THE MEDITATION BOOK OF
LIGHT AND COLOUR

by the same author

Colour Healing Manual
The Complete Colour Therapy Programme
ISBN 978 1 84819 165 5
eISBN 978 0 85701 131 2

of related interest

A Sensory Journey
Meditations on Scent for Wellbeing
Jennifer Peace Rhind
Card Set
ISBN 978 1 84819 153 2

Principles of Reflexology
What it is, how it works, and what it can do for you
Nicola Hall
Part of the Discovering Holistic Health series
ISBN 978 1 84819 137 2
eISBN 978 0 85701 108 4

Principles of Reiki
What it is, how it works, and what it can do for you
Kajsa Krishni Boräng
Foreword by Wanja Twan
Part of the Discovering Holistic Health series
ISBN 978 1 84819 138 9
eISBN 978 0 85701 109 1

Principles of the Alexander Technique
What it is, how it works, and what it can do for you
2nd edition
Jeremy Chance
Foreword by Dr David Garlick
Part of the Discovering Holistic Health series
ISBN 978 1 84819 128 0
eISBN 978 0 85701 105 3

THE MEDITATION BOOK OF LIGHT AND COLOUR

PAULINE WILLS

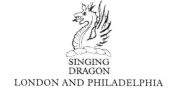

SINGING
DRAGON
LONDON AND PHILADELPHIA

Illustrations (Figures 2.1–9.1) by Rodney Paull reproduced with permission from Little, Brown Book Group.

First published in 2014
by Singing Dragon
an imprint of Jessica Kingsley Publishers
73 Collier Street
London N1 9BE, UK
and
400 Market Street, Suite 400
Philadelphia, PA 19106, USA

www.singingdragon.com

Library of Congress Cataloging in Publication Data
Wills, Pauline.
  The meditation book of light and colour / Pauline Wills.
    pages cm
  Includes index.
  ISBN 978-1-84819-202-7 (alk. paper)
  1. Color--Therapeutic use. 2. Light, Colored. 3. Phototherapy. I. Title. II. Title: Meditation book of light
and color.
  RZ414.6.W555 2014
  615.8'312--dc23
                            2013048146s

British Library Cataloguing in Publication Data
A CIP catalogue record for this book is available from the British Library

ISBN 978 1 84819 202 7
eISBN 978 0 85701 162 6

Printed and bound in Great Britain

*This book is dedicated to our wonderful friends
and neighbours Nick and Jan Nolan.*

*Special thanks to Patricia Jackson BA (Hons)
for her careful editing of the manuscript.*

CONTENTS

INTRODUCTION

I am writing this seated in my garden, on a beautiful sunny day, beneath a deep blue sky. Looking around me I see the many colours of nature, some subtle, some vibrant, and try to feel which of them I need to absorb for my well-being. As a colour practitioner I have become sensitive to colour and normally know which ones I need at any particular time to keep me in optimum health.

Colour surrounds us constantly. We can experience it in the rainbow which arcs across the sky as the sun appears after a storm, and from crystals that grow in earth's darkness and reveal their colour when brought into the daylight: such crystals have been used worldwide for centuries as a tool for healing. In certain latitudes we can witness the wonder of colour through the incredible display of polar lights known as the aurora borealis (northern lights) or the aurora australis (southern lights) – atomic energies from the sun interacting with earth's magnetism to create varicoloured patches and columns of light dancing across the sky.

The passing seasons bring us a continuous change in nature's colours – soft spring green foliage gradually moving to darker greens and then to autumnal shades of orange, yellow, red and brown. Take a moment to examine a plant's green leaves, or the petals of a red rose: you will discover that each petal or leaf has its own subtle variations of its basic colour.

Our own choice of colour is displayed in our home. If you are reading this in your home, ask yourself why you have chosen the colours of the room in which you are sitting. Is it because they are fashionable, because they are your favourite colours, or because they created the atmosphere needed for the use of that particular room? We can ask the same question of the clothes we wear. Normally we choose to wear either the season's fashionable colours, ones appropriate for our job, or hues and shades of colours which enhance our skin tone. The latter can be psychologically therapeutic because if we look good we feel good. But when we grow sensitive to colour's vibrational energy, we begin to select the colours that we need to keep us in optimum health. We may not particularly like or look good in these particular colours, but each has its own specific frequency which we may need.

We are essentially beings of light and therefore need the spectrum of colours which constitute light for our well-being. The scientific eye of aura imaging photography gives us proof of what visionaries have always claimed – that each of us is encircled and interpenetrated by a constantly changing interplay of coloured light, our electromagnetic field, or aura, which is a manifestation of our thoughts, emotions and physical condition.

Our aura consists of seven layers which interpenetrate with each other. These layers are: the physical body; the etheric body; the emotional body; the mental body; the higher mental (our higher consciousness); the causal body and the bodyless body (our true self, the part of us that is eternal). Because the colours in our aura result from our thoughts, feelings and spiritual understanding, they are constantly changing, and because these layers interpenetrate, if one layer is vibrating to the wrong frequency, it affects all the others. When we are unwell, the aura can be devoid of certain colours or the colours are in the wrong place: then we can see the truth of the saying that 'he/she is off colour'. The darker shades of a colour which appear in the aura are usually due to negative emotions. For example, a dark shade of red signifies anger while dark green signifies envy. The clear colours of the spectrum depict positive traits: a clear red is indicative of love, and the more this veers towards the lighter shade of pink, the more unconditional that love becomes; clear spectral green indicates a state of balance. If our thoughts and emotions are negative they create blockages in the energy channels (or nadis) which constitute the etheric layer of the aura. If these blockages are not cleared they can manifest as a physical disease. Using colour can help to clear energy blocks and assist a person to find and deal with the cause of the blockage. If the cause is not dealt with then the nadis again become blocked. (More information on the aura and its changing colours can be found in my book *The Colour Healing Manual*.[1])

There are many ways in which we can introduce colour into ourselves – through our environment, the clothes we wear, the food we eat and through light. If working with coloured clothes then white should be worn underneath because mixing two different colours will produce yet another colour. For example, if you wear a blue dress over yellow underwear the colour you receive will be green. Treating the body with coloured light is a very powerful therapy, but it should be used only by a properly qualified practitioner. Colour is a complementary therapy, which

1   Wills, P. (2013) *Colour Healing Manual: The Complete Colour Therapy Programme*. London: Singing Dragon.

means it can complement allopathic medicine, not replace it. If you are suffering from any kind of ill health, it is always advisable to seek medical advice.

Another way of introducing colour into ourselves is through meditation and colour breathing.

Meditation takes us on a very personal journey and it can be used in many ways. Like any journey that we undertake, it has its pitfalls and frustrations, but these can aid our learning and give us strength to continue in our quest. Meditation employs techniques that help us to transcend the physical mind and reach higher levels of consciousness where we begin to realise our true self. It also helps to improve our concentration, relieve stress and slow down our metabolism. In the busy and stressful world in which we live, all of these elements are very important for our well-being. As our body affects our mind, so our mind affects our body. Practising colour meditation brings all the above benefits and also increases our awareness of and sensitivity to particular colours, developing in us an intuitive knowledge of the colours we need at any given time to help keep our body in optimum health. Anyone working as a colour practitioner knows how very important it is to develop colour awareness and sensitivity.

Focusing on the breath is a widely practised meditation technique. It has been claimed to be the best tool for meditation because the breath is always with us. Using colour with breathing allows us to direct colour to the part of the body where it is needed or to an individual chakra which is lacking in colour. When practising the colour breathing exercises, if you are doing these at home, make sure that the room that you are in is well ventilated. If it is a warm, sunny day, open the window. When inhaling, we breathe in prana or life-force. Prana encompasses seven varieties, each of which vibrates to the frequency of one of the spectral colours. When we work with colour breathing, we visualise inhaling the colour we feel we need. We can either imagine the colour saturating our whole being or we can mentally direct the colour to the part of the body where we feel it is needed. When working with this technique, visualise red, orange and yellow entering the body through the feet, green entering horizontally at heart level and turquoise, blue, indigo, violet and magenta entering through the top of the head. Aim to make the inhalation the same length as the exhalation, allowing the breath to be slow and smooth. If at any time during colour breathing exercises you become breathless or giddy, immediately resume normal breathing.

It can be helpful to keep a record of the ways in which the colour or colours that you have worked with have affected you. If you have been practising regularly over a period of several months, it can be very interesting to look back over your notes to see how you have progressed. If you feel that you have not done too well, don't get disheartened. Remember practice makes perfect and it can take longer for some of us than for others.

When working with the exercises given in this book, it is important to practise regularly in order to gain the maximum benefit. Like any discipline, the more one works at it, the greater the results. The mind can create many reasons for not practising, so in the beginning keeping to a routine may seem quite hard.

Try to practise at the same time each day. This will establish a habit – preferably an enjoyable one. It is so easy to start the day with good intentions, promising to practise the visualisations and colour breathing exercises as soon as breakfast is over and you have space for yourself. You then realise that there is shopping to do, and other chores – or maybe you have to be at work by a certain time... And so, the end of the day comes and you are then too tired to practise... Anyway, the end of the day is not a good time because, if you are tired, there is a great temptation to fall asleep... So, the setting aside of a regular time each day is important: apart from establishing a discipline, it creates a space, a space for yourself.

In the stressful and noisy world in which we live, we all need to find space for ourselves. Initially, this involves making time each day to be alone to do the things we enjoy and to nourish ourselves in whatever way we feel is appropriate. This space can be established anywhere quiet, where we can be alone without interruption. It can be in the garden, the countryside, the park or a quiet and peaceful place in our own homes. What is important is that you try to select the same place each day. It is important because you will gradually build up harmonious and peaceful vibrations in this place and these will help you to work more easily with the meditations and colour breathing exercises. If your chosen place is in your home, you may like to have a candle, flowers or a variety of coloured crystals there. These all help to make the place very harmonious and personal to you.

If you are new to meditation and colour breathing, you will most probably find that your mind frequently wanders from what you are practising to other things that you have to do. This happens to all of us, even those who have been practising meditation and visualisation for some time. Never get annoyed or frustrated but, each time your attention strays, gently bring it back to the task in hand. Gradually, over a period of time, your mind will become used to concentrating and not wander so frequently.

Each chapter in this book will introduce a colour, explain what the colour can be used for and then give appropriate colour breathing and meditation exercises. If you feel particularly drawn towards a colour, then work with that colour. Alternatively, you may wish to explore a different colour each day. A simple dowsing technique will also be explained, to enable you to ascertain the colour you need at any given time – though it is not necessary to use this. Another way of using colour is through the chakras or energy centres. Each chakra vibrates to a specific colour, and in the appropriate chapter, a short explanation of the chakra's relevance will be given. (For those interested, an in-depth discussion of the chakras may be found in *The Colour Healing Manual.*[2])

If you are a colour practitioner you can give your clients a colour breathing or meditation exercise to work with for six days, the colour being the one most beneficial for their condition. After that period of time the overall colour needed may have changed.

I trust that working with the exercises given in this book will bring you great joy and an optimum state of health.

2   Wills, P. (2013) *Colour Healing Manual: The Complete Colour Therapy Programme.* London: Singing Dragon.

CHAPTER 1

LIGHT

You may ask why working with light is so important and why it is the opening chapter to this book. The reason is that the light that allows us to perceive the world around us radiates from the sun by day and is reflected by the moon at night. This light provides us with warmth and interacts with our molecular structure, making it vital for our well-being. Encompassed within this light are the colours of the spectrum (the colours whose vibrations make them visible to our eyes). One way of experiencing these colours is to pass light through a prism. The prism will refract the light to produce the colours of the spectrum. These colours we find displayed by nature and in the many forms of art. We use them in our homes and in the clothes we wear. Therefore they constantly surround us by day and pervade our dreams at night.

Sometimes it can be difficult to feel what colour we need. When this happens, we can work with meditations on light because light contains all the spectral colours and our body will take from the light the colour that it needs to bring it back or to keep it in optimum health. This can be likened to taking a multivitamin tablet when we are not sure which vitamins we really need. Obviously it is far better to take the vitamin which we are lacking. This also applies to working with the colour which we need.

With the advent of sophisticated scientific instruments, scientists in the USA have been able to record a very subtle energy that permeates all space and interconnects with all objects in the universe. This subtle energy field has been named the 'web of light' and 'the Divine Matrix' and in esoteric circles this subtle energy is known as the ether.

Because we individuals are a microcosm of the macrocosm, we too are surrounded by this web of light. It is present in the etheric layer of the aura, which is made up of energy channels through which light flows. It is the intersection of these light channels which form the major and minor chakras and the acupuncture points. These are the gateways through which light enters our bodies. If our bodies are energised the nadis stand upright like the branches on a tree but if they lack energy they droop like a flower that we have forgotten to water. By working with light through meditation and breathing exercises we are able to re-energise the nadis and increase our energy levels.

The meditations and breathing exercises given can be worked with at any time but it would be preferable to work with them early morning because we then re-energise ourselves in readiness for the day ahead. Work with the breathing exercise and just one of the meditations. The meditations can be alternated daily or you may find that you relate better to just one of these in which case you can work with this on a regular basis.

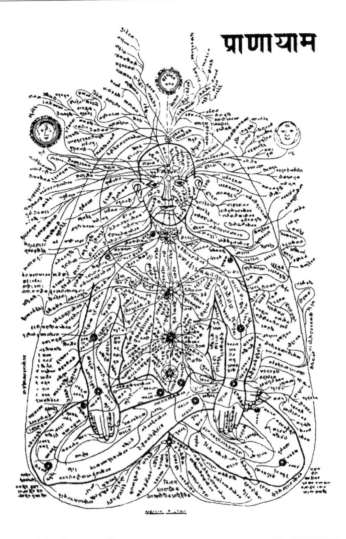

FIGURE 1.1: ANCIENT SANSKRIT DIAGRAM OF THE ENERGY CHANNELS THAT SURROUND THE PHYSICAL BODY

BREATHING IN LIGHT

Sitting in your chosen place, either on a chair or on the floor, make sure that your spine is straight and your chest open. If you are sitting on a chair, place both feet on the floor and your hands with palms down on your knees. If you are sitting on the floor, you can sit either with crossed legs or with your legs straight in front of you. Again place your hands palms down on your knees. If you are sitting on the floor, you can sit against a wall to support your back.

Gently close your eyes and bring your concentration into your breath. First, breathe in to a count of five and out to a count of five. Do this for several minutes in order to still your mind from ever-bombarding thoughts and to relax your body.

When you are ready, imagine the space that surrounds you filled with tiny brilliant white specks of dancing, vibrating light. On your next inhalation breathe in these specks of vibrating light and see them filling every part of your body. As you breathe out, allow this light to flow into the energy channels that surround you. With each inhalation, experience your body becoming more and more filled with pulsating light, and with each exhalation, see the energy channels becoming so energised that they lift up towards the light of the sun. If there is a part of your body where you are experiencing discomfort, visualise this energising white light accumulating here and bringing it back into harmony. Continue to breathe in this pulsating light for as long as you feel comfortable with it. When you are ready, breathe in, bringing your arms up over your head in order to stretch the whole of your body. As you breathe out, bring your arms back to your sides. Repeat this twice more before opening your eyes.

TRANSFERRING LIGHT

Start this exercise by taking a few normal breaths, allowing your concentration to be centred in the breath. Then place all ten fingers lightly on your solar plexus. Exhale deeply to rid the lungs of stale air.

In a relaxed manner, inhale slowly, deeply and softly. During this inhalation, imagine the white light entering your nostril, moving downwards into your solar plexus and passing into your fingertips. Slowly, and without strain, exhale. Repeat six to eight times.

When you have completed the inhalations and visualised your fingers filled with white light, retain the breath while moving your fingers to the place where there is pain or discomfort.

Exhaling slowly, imagine the white light flowing from your fingers into the chosen part of your body. When the exhalation is complete, hold the breath while you return your fingers to your solar plexus.

Repeat from the inhalation for as long as you feel it is necessary.

MEDITATIONS WITH LIGHT

THE CHALICE MEDITATION

Sit in your chosen place and relax your body and mind.

Imagine that you are sitting in a glass bulb-shaped chalice. This chalice is wide at the bottom and narrow at the top, similar to a brandy glass. The way in which it has been made enables it to reflect all the colours of the rainbow. As the light passes through the glass, the space between you and the chalice becomes filled with red, orange, yellow, green, turquoise, blue, indigo, violet and magenta, colours which are constantly dancing and playing with each other. The chalice is strong and forms a protective web around you and its colours of ethereal light represent your aura.

Looking up to the opening at the top of the chalice, visualise a shaft of white light flooding into the top of your head and resembling a waterfall of light as it flows down to permeate every cell and atom of your physical body. As this waterfall of light flows so it fills you with energy, joy and a great sense of well-being. Continue to work with this for as long as you like.

Before ending this, spend a little time meditating on this light and the feeling that it has given you.

To end, slowly increase your inhalation and exhalation and slowly open your eyes.

WINTER

Sitting in your chosen place, relax your body and mind, making sure that you spine is straight before closing your eyes.

It is winter, and the newly fallen snow lies crisp and white upon the ground, creating a blanket of stillness and silence. The bare branches of trees and stems of plants look stark against its brilliance and are bowed down beneath its weight. Small creatures have hibernated to dream of the advent of spring. Those birds that have chosen not to migrate search for food in order to survive.

In meditating upon this scene search for what it is able to teach you. White is the colour of illumination, purity and innocence; of chastity, holiness, sacredness and redemption. When it is worn by a bride, it signifies the change from single into married status. When used for funerals, it represents the death of the physical body, making way for re-birth into a new life. White is also the colour of light, of pranic energy which we need in order to energise our bodies and to sustain life.

Winter is a time when change is taking place within nature. All that which has decayed is undergoing transformation within the silence and darkness of the earth.

Do we as human beings likewise have our seasons? Can times of fruitlessness and desolation in our life be likened to winter and can these states be indicative to change – the breaking down into chaos in preparation for a new order to be established? Can winter likewise be an opportunity for us to slow down, to hibernate in our own way to allow our own energies to be restored and revitalised? All living things take time to sleep so that their energies may be recharged.

As you meditate upon this winter scene, try to ascertain what it is saying to you. Remember that this season of the year is a preparation for spring; for re-birth and transformation. Can this time of the year be likened to the fourth stage in life, namely old age? Is this a preparation for the transformation and re-birth that death accomplishes? Or is it a time for letting go of old habits and things that we no longer resonate to. These can rob us of our vital energy.

When you feel ready, bring your concentration back to your physical body, increase your inhalation and exhalation and then gently open your eyes.

If you feel that it would be advantageous, you can now work with one of the pranic breathing exercises to recharge your body.

THE MOUNTAIN POOL

Go to your chosen place and, if you feel that it is appropriate for you, light a candle. Sitting quietly, either on a chair or on the floor, bring your concentration to your breath. Slowly breathe in to five and out to five. This will help to relax your body and quieten your mind.

When you feel ready, imagine yourself sitting by a clear mountain pool. It is a warm day with just a slight breeze which makes tiny ripples on the surface of the pool. You are surrounded by mountains, the higher ones capped with the last of winter's snow. You are alone in the silence of this beautiful landscape. Alone to dream your dreams and to look at yourself.

Looking into the pool you can see the bottom which has a few small rounded stones nestling amongst the larger flat mountainous rock. Taking off your shoes, put your feet into the clear cool water. At first it feels cold but as you get used to this you feel the energy of the water slowly creeping up your legs. Water is liquid light and has its own cellular memory. Because this pool has never been polluted, its molecular structure forms the most beautiful flower patterns.

If it feels right for you, immerse yourself into the water and swim amongst its vibrant energies.

Feel the energy of the water removing any tension that may be present and replacing this with a sense of peace and relaxation. Allow the water to re-energise your whole being and to remove any discomfort you may be experiencing. In the silence, contemplate your life and ask yourself what, if any, changes you need to make in order to become more fulfilled and healthy within yourself. Ask to be intuitively shown the best way to bring about these changes. If you are at a crossroads in your life, seek to find the correct path to take. Sometimes it takes a great deal of courage to follow the path that we intuitively know is right for us because this path can present difficulties which require courage to face.

When you are ready, come out of the water and lie down beneath a brilliant blue sky. Feel the warmth of the sun upon you and in the silence, contemplate the refreshing, energising power of water and what it feels like to be submerged in the purity of liquid light. Think about the questions you may have asked yourself and listen for an answer. This may not come immediately but when the time is right, you will be shown the best path for you.

When you are ready, slowly increase your inhalation and exhalation and then gently open your eyes. Remain sitting for a few minutes to think about the experiences you may have had.

CHAPTER 2

RED

Red is a vibrant and warm colour and sits next to infra-red on the electromagnetic spectrum. It has the longest wavelength and lowest energy of all visible light. The energy of a colour is determined by how far apart the energy packages, or quanta, are. In red they are the furthest apart of all the colours. As with every colour, red has its own spectrum which ranges from very deep to very pale. The bright translucent shades of a colour relate to its positive aspects, while the dark and dingy shades display its negative side. In most cultures red stands for the masculine principle. It is symbolic of the sun and all the gods attributed to war.

The word red comes from the old English *read*. Further back in history, the word can be traced to the Proto-Germanic *rautbaz* and the Proto-Indo European root *reudh*. The varying shades of this colour derived their name from their source. Both cinnabar and vermilion are ancient names for a red crystalline form of mercuric sulphide. Crimson and carmine derive from the Latin *kermesius*, the name of the dye extracted from the kermes insect. Alizarin is one of the compounds found in the root of the *rubia tinctoria* plant, and this gives its red colouring to a paint and dye known as Rose Madder.

Physically red is linked to the circulatory system, to the heart and to fertility (the reason an Indian bride wears a red sari on her wedding day). In human psychology red is associated with emotions that 'stir the blood', including anger, passion and love.

Red is a good colour for warming the body. This is why we wear red gloves and socks in the winter and why in Victorian times red nightshirts were popular. Red also helps to counteract infections because it increases the blood supply to an infected area, allowing the white corpuscles found in blood to deal with the invading bacteria. (For the same reason an infected finger was put into hot water.)

Because red is a powerful, energising and stimulating colour, it is not advisable for those suffering from anxiety, emotional disturbances, high blood pressure or heart problems to use it. Also, it is not a good colour to use in a bedroom, unless you wish to spend restless nights. Small quantities of red are good in a dining room because red can aid digestion. But use too much red and you could end up with indigestion!

THE BASE CHAKRA

Red is associated with the base chakra, the energy centre which is situated at the end of the spine (the coccyx). The Sanskrit name given to this chakra is *Muladhara*, meaning root or foundation. This chakra is the foundation upon which we build our lives. In books on subtle anatomy it is depicted as a circle with four outer red petals. Inside the circle is a yellow square representing the earth element and, like the earth, the square shape is solid and stable making it a perfect foundation upon which to start any spiritual journey. Inside the square, symbols of the chakra's many attributes are displayed. These take the forms of gods and goddesses, animals, etc.

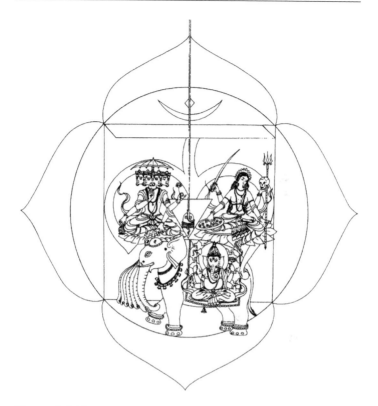

FIGURE 2.1: THE BASE CHAKRA

The parts of the body affected by the base chakra are the legs, feet, bones, large intestine, spine and nervous system. The associated endocrine glands are the testes.

When this centre is functioning fully, it gives a person a strong will to live on the physical plane. He/she is filled with vitality and energy, nothing is too much trouble, and the whole of life becomes an adventure. If, however, this centre is not functioning to its full potential, a person's energy levels will decline, there will be a lack of enthusiasm for life, and daily work will tend to become burdensome. Depression and lack of confidence may well follow.

One way in which you can test your own chakras is through a simple technique derived from kinesiology.

First, join the thumb and first finger of your left hand to form a circle. Next, place the first finger of your right hand inside that circle. When you have done this, bring your concentration to the chakra you wish to test and, keeping your mind focused on this centre, try to break the left hand circle by pressing the first finger of your right hand down onto it. If you are able to break the circle then the chakra is weak or devoid of energy. If you are unable to break the circle then the chakra is strong.

Another way of checking your chakras is by dowsing. To do this you will need a pendulum. A pendulum can be made of wood, crystal or metal. If you do not wish to buy a manufactured pendulum you can use a pendant on a chain, or a ring with a piece of cotton or string threaded through it. If you choose to work with a pendulum, it is important to possess your own. Likewise, a pendant or ring should be yours.

If you buy a pendulum, it should be cleansed from any old or negative vibrations. The simplest way of doing this is to leave it in salt water overnight then wash it the following morning under running water. When you have cleansed it, carry it around in your pocket for a couple of weeks to enable it to become permeated with your own energy.

Learning to work with a pendulum takes time and patience. The first step is to discover your 'yes' and 'no' response. To do this, hold the pendulum approximately 15 cm away from your solar plexus and mentally ask it to indicate your 'yes'. It will respond by swinging either clockwise or anti-clockwise or in a horizontal or diagonal line. Now ask it to indicate your 'no'. It will respond by swinging in another direction. Once established, these responses should always be the same for you.

As before, bring your attention to the chakra you wish to test, then ask 'Is this chakra strong?' or 'Is my [name of the chakra] strong?' The pendulum will move either in your 'yes' or your 'no' direction. Remember that the pendulum will answer only 'yes' or 'no', so you need to make your questions very precise.

Initially, dowsing can produce doubts in our mind and we may wonder if the information we have collected is correct. The lesson we need to learn from this is trust. Also, when dowsing for ourselves we have to be totally detached, otherwise we can influence the pendulum to give the answer we wish to hear.

Some of the physical disorders arising from a malfunctioning base chakra are spinal and leg problems, testicular disorders, haemorrhoids and inhibited rejuvenation of red blood cells.

BREATHING IN RED

Sitting in your chosen place, either on a chair or on the floor, bring your concentration into your breath. Do not try to control the breath but just be aware of your gentle inhalation and exhalation. With each exhalation feel your body gently relaxing and your mind becoming quiet and still.

When you feel relaxed and at peace, bring your concentration back to the breath and gradually increase your inhalation and exhalation to a count of eight. If you find that this is uncomfortable, reduce the count to five or six.

On your next inhalation, visualise a beam of red light coming from the earth into your base chakra. As you breathe out, allow this light to radiate into your aura, down both legs and back to the earth. Practise this for as long as it feels right for you. Then allow your breath to return to its normal pattern and, sitting quietly, let yourself be aware of any changes this colour has brought about in you.

CHANNELLING RED LIGHT THROUGH THE HANDS

Sitting comfortably, place your hands on your solar plexus. The solar plexus is where the solar plexus chakra (yellow) is situated, but the solar plexus is also a part of our anatomy which is frequently used for breathing techniques and for transferring energy, so here we are not working with the solar plexus chakra but with our anatomy. On your next inhalation, visualise a beam of red light coming into your solar plexus from the earth. As you exhale allow this light to flood into your hands. Continue to breathe in red and discharge it into your hands until they become infused with red light. Now place your hands on any part of your body that feels cold or where you may have a minor infection. If you are suffering leg problems, place your hands on the part of the leg where the problem lies.

At the end of this exercise, place your hands on your thighs, return to normal breathing and sit quietly for a few minutes, contemplating this colour's effect upon you.

MEDITATIONS WITH THE COLOUR RED

MEDITATION ON THE RED GLOW OF A FIRE

Sitting in your chosen place, visualise yourself walking towards a small country cottage on a cold winter's evening. All is peaceful and quiet. Frost on the grass and trees sparkles in the moonlight. The wind blows chill, penetrating the clothes you are wearing.

Upon reaching the front door of your cottage, open it with your key and walk through into the hall, closing the door behind you. Removing your outer clothing, you feel a sense of relief at being away from the cold night air. Walking from the hall into the sitting room, you find a blazing log fire burning in the grate. Sitting down in front of the fire you allow its warmth to thaw your chilled hands and feet. The only light in the room is provided by the fire, which creates gently moving shadows upon the walls and ceiling. As you sit looking into the fire, be aware of the various shades of red produced by the flames and watch how the flames dance with each other. Visualise the warmth from the fire spreading from your hands and feet through your entire body. Be conscious of your whole being as it is engulfed in the varying shades of red. Meditate upon the effect that this colour is having on the various parts of your body. Do you feel that the effect is more prevalent in particular areas? Do you feel energised by it? Is it a colour that you enjoy, or one that you would prefer not to be surrounded by? What is the overall feeling that this colour gives you?

When you feel that you have considered your response to this colour sufficiently, slowly begin to increase your inhalation and exhalation and, when you are ready, gently open your eyes.

MEDITATION ON A FLOWER

Find a red flower and put it into water or, if you have a garden with a red flower in bloom, you can sit in front of the flower. Look at the flower and observe how delicate and perfectly shaped the petals are. Notice the differences in the formation of each petal and the varying shades of red within them. If you have the flower in a vase, take it and place it on the palm of your left hand. Hold the palm of your right hand about three to four inches above it. If you are working with a flower that is growing in a garden, gently place your hands around it. Close your eyes and, bringing the whole of your concentration into your hands, try to feel through them the vibration of the colour. After a few moments, return the cut flower to its vase, or gently release the garden flower, and gaze at it for a few moments. Close your eyes again and try to visualise it. Visualise the shape and the colour. Try to feel and become one with that colour. If any part of your body feels cold, imagine the colour flowing to that area of the body. Feel the cold being replaced with warmth. Now visualise this colour flowing into the base chakra. See this chakra being brought into balance and, at the same time, feel the colour red earthing and grounding you.

When you are ready, gently open your eyes and allow yourself a few moments of reflection before ending this meditation session.

MEDITATION ON A RED ROSE

Close your eyes and visualise yourself sitting in front of a partially opened red rose. Note the different shades of red the rose displays and the softness and delicacy of its petals.

As you contemplate the rose, it slowly starts to grow in size until it is large enough for you to crawl into it and lie down at its centre. As you rest comfortably on the bed of soft petals, the sun's rays play upon their outer surface, creating a soft red light that floods the flower's heart. This colour surrounds and interpenetrates all aspects of your being. It creates a pleasantly warm feeling and its vibrant energy starts to invigorate you.

Look at this colour until your eyes start to become tired, then close them and try to visualise the colour red before your closed eyes. When you have achieved this, use your imagination to take this colour to any part of your body that feels cold. Visualise the part of your body that you are working with suffused in red light, then visualise this light increasing the blood supply to this area, resulting in a gradual increase of warmth to the point where the chosen part of your body feels quite hot.

If you feel that your base chakra needs energising, take the colour there. See the colour swirling around the chakra, revitalising all the parts of the body associated with it.

Now spend a little time meditating upon this colour. How do you relate to it? Is it a pleasant colour to work with? Do you like or dislike it?

In your own time, crawl out from inside the flower and sit in front of it. Watch as the flower slowly shrinks back to its normal size, then gently open your eyes.

SUNRISE

Sitting in your chosen place, gently close your eyes and imagine that you are walking in the countryside just before sunrise. All is peaceful and still except for the sound of a tiny bubbling brook in the distance. The trees that line the path you are walking look black in the darkness of night and the grass seems to be devoid of colour. Before you is a grassy mound.

Upon reaching this you slowly walk to its top and sit down on the cool, soft grass. As you look towards the horizon, the sun starts to appear. Its first rays break the darkness of night like red spears, before they fan out into red's various pastel shades across the night sky.

With the advent of dawn the first cockerel awakens and its morning call rouses the birds that have been nesting in the trees, safe from any predators. The silence of night gradually becomes a melody of bird song that is slowly accompanied by the bleating of sheep and the lowing of cows. The countryside has awakened.

Looking at the various shades of red that have spread across the sky, imagine yourself becoming wrapped in a cloak encompassing all those shades. Enjoy differentiating between them and decide which of them you are particularly drawn towards.

Having chosen your favourite shade of red, visualise it becoming the dominant colour of your cloak. Try to feel what it is doing for you and meditate upon why you have chosen this particular shade of red. Is it your favourite colour, or do you feel that you need this colour? If you feel a need of it, try to determine why.

When you are ready, open your eyes and reflect for a few moments on your experience.

CHAPTER 3

ORANGE

The colour orange lies between red and yellow in the visible light spectrum at a wavelength of approximately 585–620 nm (nanometres). Orange pigments are largely in the ochre or cadmium families.

The colour was first introduced into the English as *geoluhread*, which translates into modern English as yellow-red. It was subsequently named after the orange fruit, introduced to Europe from the Sanskrit word *naranji*. The first recorded English use of orange as a named colour was in 1512, at the court of King Henry VIII. The rich, vibrant dyes that appeared in the nineteenth century were produced from the red, fleshy root of the madder flower. Today's deep luxurious shades are produced from synthetic dyes.

Orange is the symbol of feminine energy, the energy of creation. It is gentler than the dynamic, masculine energy of red but is complementary to it. It is therefore important that these two colours should work in harmony. It is a warm colour, one typical of the hot spices used in Eastern countries.

Orange is also associated with fruitfulness and sexuality. The ancient custom of adorning a bride with orange blossom was symbolic of this. In past eras the orange seeds of the pomegranate were taken as an aphrodisiac.

The colour of joy and happiness, orange enables us to create a balance between our physical and mental bodies. (Red is associated with the physical body and yellow with the intellect: the two colours when combined produce orange.) It gives freedom to thoughts and feelings and disperses heaviness, allowing the body natural, joyful movements. This makes it a good colour to use in rooms of activity and family gatherings.

Orange brings about changes in the body's biochemical structure, resulting in the dispersal of depression.

THE SACRAL CHAKRA

Orange is associated with the sacral chakra, which is situated halfway between the pubis and the navel. This chakra's Sanskrit name is *Swadisthana*, meaning 'one's own abode', and it is represented by a circle with six orange outer petals. The orange petals symbolise the chakra's association with creative, sexual energy and the joy that comes with the creation of a human form to house an incarnating soul. Inside the circle is a crescent moon representing the water element. The moon controls the ebb and flow of the oceans as well as our own emotional fluctuations. The sacral chakra is linked with the etheric layer of the aura and with the element of water, and it affects the flow of fluids in the body. This chakra becomes active at puberty, a time that can be emotionally traumatic in many young people.

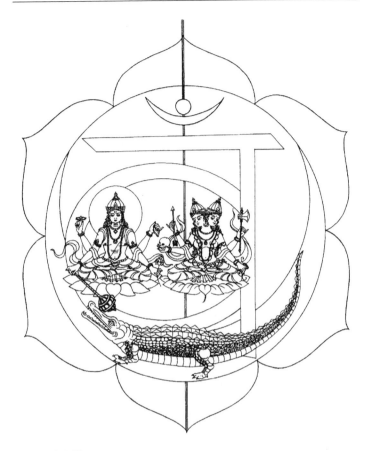

FIGURE 3.1: THE SACRAL CHAKRA

The glands and organs which *Swadisthana* influences are the skin, the reproductive organs (especially those related to a female), the kidneys, bladder and circulatory and lymphatic systems. The endocrine glands associated with it are the adrenals.

The adrenals are our 'fight or flight' glands, therefore the chakra is also emotionally linked with fear and anxiety. A chakra's colour does not necessarily mean that it just takes on the attributes of the colour; it can also take on the attributes of its element (in this case water) and the endocrine gland that it is linked with.

Some of the physical disorders that can arise from this chakra are dysfunction of the reproductive organs, intestinal complaints and bladder and kidney disorders. When this chakra is balanced, we are in touch with our emotions and trusting towards others. Too much energy here can result in an over-emotional, aggressive, over-ambitious, manipulative nature, but when the chakra is deficient in energy we can become over-sensitive, timid, resentful and distrustful.

BREATHING IN ORANGE
ENERGISING THE ABDOMINAL ORGANS WITH ORANGE

Sitting in your chosen place, gently close your eyes, bringing your concentration into your breath. Breathing normally, feel the breath entering and leaving your lungs. With each out-breath, release any tension present in the body. When you are ready, visualise a shaft of orange light rising from the earth and flowing up your legs into your sacral chakra. As you exhale, allow this colour to flow from the chakra into your abdomen and then into your aura. Focusing your attention on your sacral chakra, try to be aware of any effect this colour is having upon it. Are you able to feel this energy centre? Are you able to visualise the colour?

Continue to practise this exercise for as long as you feel is right for you. Then, when you are ready, return to normal breathing and consider whether this colour has affected you in any way.

ENERGISING THE SACRAL CHAKRA THROUGH THE BREATH

Sitting comfortably in your chosen place, slowly start to relax your body. Then, when you are ready, bring your awareness to your sacral chakra. Visualise the chakra as a deep orange chrysanthemum. As you breathe in to a count of seven or eight, visualise a shaft of deep orange light coming from the earth, up through your legs and into the chakra. As the colour comes into contact with the chrysanthemum, watch the petals start to radiate a deep, clear, orange light. Slowly breathing out to seven or eight, observe how the orange light reflects out from the petals into your abdomen. As you continue to visualise the inhalation and exhalation of this bright, clear orange, the sacral chakra is cleared of any stagnant energy and becomes energised and balanced. With practice, this exercise will help to keep all your abdominal organs healthy.

When you are ready, bring your awareness back to your physical body and, before opening your eyes, reflect on any changes this exercise has brought about within you.

MEDITATIONS WITH THE COLOUR ORANGE

VISUALISATION WITH THE COLOUR ORANGE

Sitting in your chosen place, relax your body and quieten your mind.

Visualise yourself sitting on the beach at dusk. The air is still warm from the heat of the day and the seagulls and other daytime birds have returned to their nesting place for the night. The only sound to be heard is that of the waves as they break upon the shore. Gradually synchronise your breath with the tide's ebb and flow, inhaling as the waves break and exhaling as they pull back from the shore. Turn your attention to the sun as it slowly sinks below the horizon. Its yellow rays have now turned to a deep orange, shooting like blazing arrows across the darkening sky, creating a fiery golden reflection upon the ocean beneath. These blazing orange arrows reach and enter your body, filling you with a warm, orange glow. Any depression you may have been experiencing is gently dispersed and replaced with a wonderful feeling of joy and energy. In this relaxed and uplifted state, visualise your body filling with orange light, noting the feelings this arouses within you, physically, mentally and emotionally.

When you are ready, bring your awareness back to the horizon where the sun has now set, leaving behind it the deep indigo sky of night. Feel this deep indigo wrapping you in a cloak of peace and protection before you open your eyes.

MEDITATION ON AN ORANGE

Sitting in your chosen place, hold an orange in the palms of your hands. Feel its skin, noting the variations in its texture. Look carefully at its colour to see if this is uniform throughout. Note the form that the orange has taken.

In your imagination take the orange back to its source, the tree upon which it grew and the tiny seed that produced the tree. For what purpose did the tree bear fruit: would it have been in order to reproduce itself? What would have become of the fruit had it not been picked; would it have fallen from the tree and decayed?

Mentally pass through the outer skin of the orange to its soft fleshy inside. Try to conjure up the taste of the orange, its aroma and the texture and colour of its flesh.

Picture the orange increasing in size until it encompasses you, enabling you to sit at its centre. Looking around the inside of the orange you see the small clusters of seeds – seeds which, if planted, will eventually produce new orange trees. Consider how such a small part of the orange is able to bear the blueprint for such a large tree. Think about yourself, and how a minute, fertilised ovum miraculously bears the blueprint for a human being. Is the seed within the orange its very essence? If so, what is this essence, this energy, this blueprint? Likewise, is the fertilised ovum your very essence and, if so, what does this represent to you?

Each of you will come up with a different answer to these questions, and this answer is right for you. You may not know the answer, and this is also OK. What you might contemplate here is what the essence of life means to you. Is it that divine energy that brought all things into being, whatever name you wish to give to this, or could it be something else?

Now feel the orange cloaking you in an aura of orange light. Meditate upon how this colour feels and also upon the very essence of life.

When you are ready, gently increase your inhalation and exhalation before opening your eyes.

THE GARDEN

Sitting comfortably in your chosen place, gently close your eyes and imagine that you are sitting in a garden on a warm summer's day. You can sit on a bench or on the grass, whichever you prefer. In front of you lies a flower bed bordered with marigolds in varying shades of orange. Looking at the colour of these flowers you call to mind that orange is the colour of joy and dance, for as joy lifts our spirits it encourages carefree movement, the movement of dance.

Meditate upon your life at present. Are you joyful, taking part in all the activities that you would wish, or are you experiencing sadness and depression? If the latter is true, consider what might be the cause of these negative emotions and the best way of dealing with them. At first you may find this a difficult thing to do: but remember, only by discovering and eradicating the causes of negativity in your life can you again experience that wonderful feeling of joy.

Our true nature is one of joy, and we lack this when we focus on adverse things or circumstances, thus throwing ourselves off centre. Our mind affects our body in the same way that our body affects our mind. When we are truly ourselves, allowing ourselves to be free from all negative thoughts and resolving those issues that trouble us, only then can we come back into that state of joy which is truly ours.

Now look back to an event or a place where you experienced real joy and happiness. Allow yourself to re-create these feelings so that you again experience them throughout your whole being. Each time that you feel depressed try reliving any occasion that you thoroughly enjoyed.

When you are ready, open your eyes and spend a few moments thinking about ways of creating more joy in your life.

THE TEMPLE

Going to your chosen place, lie down and bring your concentration into the breath. With each out-breath release any tension present, enabling your body and mind to go into a deep state of relaxation.

Imagine that you are lying on a soft white cloud. Very slowly, the cloud starts to take you out of the place where you are lying and up into the indigo sky of night. Passing through the night sky you marvel at the thousands of stars shining like many faceted diamonds. Gazing upon this wonderful sight you begin to hear the individual sound of each star as they combine to produce an exquisite, ever-changing harmony.

Passing through the night sky, your soft white cloud brings you into a valley and slowly lowers you to the ground. Standing up you let your eyes travel over the serene landscape with its beautiful trees and flowers until, in the distance, you notice a circular building. Slowly you walk towards it, appreciating and enjoying the myriad colours of nature that surround you.

Approaching the building you notice that there are seven steps leading up to a door. Climbing the stairs, you push the door open and walk through into a circular room. The floor is carpeted in a soft blue and the surrounding walls are white. Looking up to the ceiling you observe that it is a dome made from interlocking crystals which flood the room with a very soft white light. At the centre of the room a fountain plays.

Suddenly you are aware of a presence standing next to you. It introduces itself as the guardian of the place and invites you to approach the fountain. Then, as you reach the fountain, you are invited to step into the water. Standing in the centre of the fountain you are aware that the water showering upon you is a most vibrant shade of orange. Bathing in this liquid light, you feel any depression and anxiety being washed away and your whole being becoming flooded with a sense of joy and vitality.

When you are ready, step out of the fountain and thank its guardian for this wonderful experience. With joy and vitality flowing through you, walk back to the entrance, pass through the door and down the steps into the valley. Walk back along the valley to where your white cloud is awaiting you. Climbing onto the cloud, allow it to lift you out of the valley, up into the indigo night sky and to bring you safely back to where your body is lying.

Slowly start to increase your exhalation and inhalation, and then take some time to contemplate your experience before opening your eyes.

CHAPTER 4

YELLOW

Yellow is the colour nearest to sunlight with a wavelength of 556–589 nm. The word yellow comes from the old English *geolu* or *geolwe* which derived from the proto-Germanic word *gelwaz*.

In the English language yellow has been traditionally associated with jaundice and cowardice. This link could have arisen from sixteenth-century Spain where a person found guilty of heresy and treason was made to wear yellow. Also a coward can be said to be 'yellow-bellied' or 'yellow'. This colour is also associated with caution. The central traffic light is amber, a mixture of yellow and orange. Yellow is linked to ageing for both people and objects. Old paper turns yellow and elderly people's skins sometimes take on a yellowish tint.

In Italy the word yellow refers to crime stories. This association began when the first series of crime novels published in Italy had yellow covers. Yellow is linked with the mind and the intellect. Because it represents the power of thought and stimulates mental activity it is a good colour to have in small quantities in a place of study. It is also the colour of detachment and can therefore help us to free ourselves from obsessive thoughts, feelings and habits.

The yellow light rays carry positive magnetic currents which are inspiring and stimulating. They strengthen our nervous system and stimulate higher mentality. This colour activates the motor nerves in the physical body, thereby generating energy in the muscles.

Yellow has a beneficial effect on the skin, improving its texture, and cleansing and healing scars and other disorders such as eczema. The reason for this may be because it is the colour nearest to sunlight.

THE SOLAR PLEXUS CHAKRA

The Sanskrit name given to this chakra is *Manipura*, which means 'the jewel of the navel'. Its dominant colour is yellow. It is connected to the element of fire and the sense of sight and is ruled by the sun. The solar plexus chakra is situated just above the navel and is associated with the aura's astral or emotional layer, therefore any emotional turmoil in our lives greatly affects this centre. It is depicted as a bright yellow lotus flower with ten petals.

This is the centre of vitality in the physical body because it is where prana (the upward moving vitality) and apana (the downward moving vitality) meet, generating the heat that is necessary to support life.

The solar plexus chakra is chiefly concerned with the process of digestion and absorption. Processes and organs influenced by it are the breath, the diaphragm, the stomach, duodenum, gall bladder and liver. The endocrine gland with which it is associated is the pancreas.

Only part of the pancreas is endocrine – the part known as 'the islets of Langerhans'. This area secretes insulin, which is responsible for the metabolism of sugar.

When this chakra is balanced we have self-respect for ourselves and others. We are outgoing, cheerful, relaxed and spontaneous and experience a deep and fulfilling emotional life. When the chakra is unstable, we can be subjected to rapid mood swings. There can be a tendency towards depression, introversion, lethargy, poor digestion and abnormal eating habits.

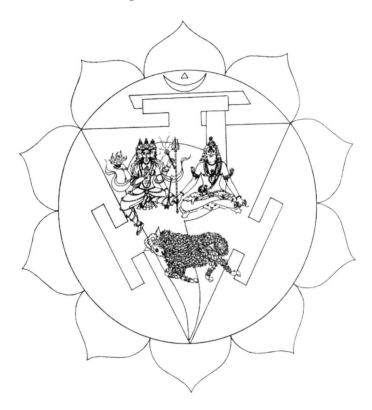

FIGURE 4.1: THE SOLAR PLEXUS CHAKRA

BREATHING IN YELLOW
ENERGISING THE SOLAR PLEXUS WITH YELLOW

Sit down in your chosen place, either on a chair or on the floor. Make sure that your spine is straight and your body relaxed.

Bring your awareness into your solar plexus. Feel and visualise the organs that are housed in this part of your body; these are the liver, stomach, pancreas and spleen. Imagine your solar plexus chakra as a bright yellow sun which is fed by the yellow shaft of light that you bring through the earth with each inhalation. As you feed your sun with yellow light, it grows and glows more brightly. You begin to feel all the organs and glands connected with this energy centre starting to radiate the warm, gentle heat of life and vitality. With each exhalation, visualise the warm bright rays from the solar plexus chakra reaching out to other parts of your body, particularly places where you may be experiencing discomfort. Allow the warmth and light to disperse any negative and unwanted energy in order that your physical body may experience vitality and health.

When you are ready, increase your inhalation and exhalation before opening your eyes.

ENERGISING THE ETHERIC AND PHYSICAL BODY WITH YELLOW

Sit down in your chosen place, either on a chair or on the floor. Make sure that your spine is straight and your body relaxed.

Bring your concentration to your solar plexus chakra. Breathing in to a count of seven, visualise a shaft of clear yellow light coming from the earth, through your feet and into your solar plexus chakra. As you exhale to a count of seven, allow this colour to radiate into your physical body and out into your aura. Feel its soothing effect upon your nervous system and its strengthening effect on your skeletal system. Visualise it entering the nadis in the etheric layer of the aura to bring more vitality into your body. Allow this colour to work on your intellect, aiding better concentration. Now imagine yourself glowing with the warmth and vitality of the sun.

As you gently inhale and exhale this colour, note any changes that are occurring within you, both physically and mentally. How do you relate to this colour? If you have chosen to keep a diary of your work with colour, note down any changes you have experienced. Every time that you work with a colour, your responses to it will vary.

When you are ready, return to normal breathing for a few seconds before opening your eyes.

MEDITATIONS WITH THE COLOUR YELLOW
DETACHMENT

Imagine yourself, on a warm summer's day, walking through a wild flower meadow. Grasses and flowers grow in abundance and bees and butterflies are enjoying the plentiful supply of nectar. Everywhere, standing tall above the grasses, bright yellow buttercups sway on slender stems. Picking a buttercup's cup-shaped flower, become aware of its five shiny petals surrounding its fine yellow stamens. Notice how delicately formed the petals are. Still holding the flower, lie down in the field and visualise these soft, yellow flowers enfolding you in a glowing yellow light. Gradually feel this colour detaching you from your family and friends, your home and personal belongings. In this state of detachment, look at any problems you may at present be experiencing and search for an appropriate solution for them. Sometimes, our problems can be similar to standing in a forest and not being able to see, for the trees, the many paths that lead out of the forest. The colour yellow can act as an air balloon that lifts us above the forest so that we can see the path we must take in order to solve our problems. In this state of detachment, where your emotions cannot influence your decisions, meditate upon any changes you need to make in order to live a fuller and more enriched life. Change can at times be difficult and challenging because it can threaten our security but, as the old saying goes, 'no change no progress'. Yellow can portray the coward within us, and this is related to our reluctance to make changes in our life. But in this meditation we are using yellow's stimulating energy and positivity to help us become who we truly are by making the necessary lifestyle changes.

Quietly meditate upon how you are reacting to the yellow light that is surrounding you and be aware of how it is stimulating you to look at any changes you need to make in your life in order to move forward.

EVENING

A hot sultry day has given way to a light, soothing evening breeze. The rush of the day has abated and peace starts to descend upon the earth.

Visualise yourself walking along a soft, sandy beach. The only noise is the sound of the waves as they roll across the sand and then withdraw back to the ocean. Feel the softness of the sand beneath your feet. Compared with the heat of the day the sand feels pleasantly cool and refreshing to walk on. Finding a small cove, lie down on the soft sand

and allow the stresses of the day to leave your body. As your body and mind start to relax, visualise the golden yellow colour of the sand entering your body through your feet. With each slow intake of breath, the colour rises up your legs, into your abdomen and chest, and finally into your head, bathing you in a beautiful, soft golden yellow light. As you become relaxed and detached from all that surrounds you, meditate upon the day that is slowly passing. Look at any negativity that you may have encountered, any emotional upsets or depression. Try to realise the cause of these and consider how you can prevent them re-occurring. Try to see them as a learning curve, treating them as experiences that teach you how to become a more mature and contented person. Learn to laugh at your mistakes rather than looking at them in a negative way because there is no way in which we can change mistakes; we can only learn from them.

Now meditate upon all the positive things that have happened. Congratulate yourself on your successes and acknowledge all the good things that you have achieved. So often we are apt to dwell on our mistakes and not congratulate ourselves on our achievements. Look forward to tomorrow, viewing this as a clean page in your book of life, and endeavour to make it a happy day in which you achieve all the things that you set out to do.

Bringing your awareness back to your physical body, feel the warm glow that this golden colour is giving you and be aware of how relaxed and peaceful you feel.

Take time to meditate upon these thoughts, then, when you are ready, slowly start to increase your inhalation and exhalation before opening your eyes.

STIMULATING YOUR INTELLECT

This is a good meditation to start your day with or before starting any intellectual pursuit. Yellow is the colour of sunshine, of sunflowers, daffodils and ripe corn. A bright yellow is the colour of the intellect and can be used for mental stimulation and for helping us to think more clearly.

Sitting quietly in your chosen place, visualise a golden yellow sun shining in the vastness of the cosmos. Realise how very small we are in this vast, ever-growing universe in which we live. But also realise how unique each of us is as a human being – every one of us being given our own talents and purpose for life on this earth.

As you concentrate upon the sun, feel its warmth upon you and allow its light to disperse any negativity that you may be feeling. Visualise its life-affirming rays beaming gently down upon your head and filling your brain with a rich, golden yellow. This colour stimulates your brain, sharpens your intellect and removes any confusion, tiredness or haziness, allowing you to think more clearly. It allows you to see situations in a different light and gives you new ideas connected to your daily tasks. As you visualise this colour circulating around your head, allow your mind to quieten in order to listen to your intuition. Stay with this meditation for as long as you wish, then gently increase your inhalation and exhalation before opening your eyes.

This is a good colour to meditate with when you are seeking answers to a problem or a life situation, being confident that when the time is right, an answer will be given. Answers can come through a friend, through a book you are reading or through sitting quietly in a meditative state.

CHAPTER 5

GREEN

Green is in the middle of the colour spectrum with a wavelength of approximately 520–570 nm. The word comes from the old English word *grene*, or, in its older form, *groeni*. *Groeni* is closely associated to the old English verb *growan* (to grow) and derives from Western Germanic and Scandinavian languages.

Green, a colour frequently used in describing foliage and the sea, has become a symbol of environmentalism. Greens, together with blues and purples, are often called cool colours in contrast to the warm colours of red, yellow and orange.

Green provides a sense of balance in all aspects of ourselves. It has the strength to integrate the intuitive right and intellectual left hemispheres of the brain. It is a very restful colour for the eyes because the eyes focus green light almost exactly on the retina. Anyone working long hours with a computer could benefit their eyes by spending time amongst the varied greens of nature. Green also has antiseptic properties – the reason why green malachite was used as a protective eyeliner in ancient Egypt. The colour's soothing quality causes some theatres to name a backstage room the 'green room', for actors awaiting their cue or entertaining friends – and part of the benefit of a country walk is the calming effect of the surrounding greenery.

Successful gardeners, cooperating with nature's life-giving aspects, are said to have 'green fingers'.

In the natural world, green is the colour of life, found in the new foliage of spring and the mature foliage of summer. It is balanced by the duller greens found in decaying vegetation. Green's negative attributes are associated with envy and jealousy. An envious person may well be labelled a 'green-eyed monster'. It is also associated with nausea and sickness – a physically ill person being described as looking 'green around the gills'.

THE HEART CHAKRA

Green is associated with the heart chakra, which is situated slightly to the right of the physical heart. Its Sanskrit name is *Anahata*, meaning the unstruck or unbeaten sound. All the sound in the universe is produced by striking objects together. This sets up vibrations or sound waves. But the sound that comes from beyond this material world, known as the primordial sound, is the source of all sound, and is the vibration of ultimate reality. This, the highest of vibrations, is said to be that of unconditional love, and so is connected to the heart chakra.

The heart chakra is symbolised by a green lotus flower with 12 green petals. At its centre is an interlaced triangle characterising the union of opposites. The upward-pointing triangle represents solar energy and fire and embodies the masculine principle. The downward-pointing triangle is linked with the moon, water and the feminine principle and is associated with the element of air and the sense of touch.

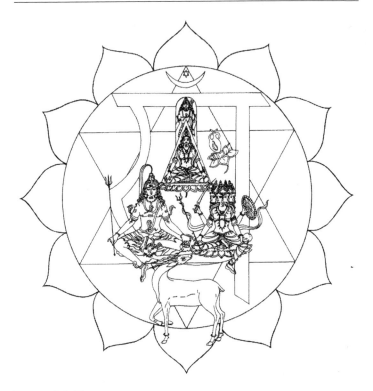

FIGURE 5.1: THE HEART CHAKRA

On a physical level, *Anahata* is associated with the heart and circulatory system, the lungs and respiratory system, the immune system and the arms and hands. The endocrine gland attributed to it is the thymus, which plays an important role in the body's immune system.

This is the centre through which we love. Love can be expressed on many levels. It can be purely selfish, demanding and constricting, or it can be compassionate and caring. The more open this centre is, the greater our capacity to extend undemanding spiritual love. When we are able to transform personal desires and passions into a love that encompasses our fellow human beings, animals and nature, the energies from the solar plexus chakra are raised into the heart chakra. It is through the heart chakra that we make cords to connect with those with whom we have a love relationship. When this centre is open, we can perceive the beauty and spiritual love in our fellow human beings. Its awakening brings a greater sensitivity to the sense of touch and a detachment from material possessions.

When the heart chakra's energy is balanced, we are compassionate, have a desire to nurture others and have an understanding of unconditional love. Too much heart energy can make us demanding, moody and depressed: but if the chakra is deficient in energy we can be indecisive, have a fear of being rejected and need constant reassurance.

Some of the physical disorders that can be associated with the heart chakra are high blood pressure, heart and lung problems and asthma.

BREATHING IN GREEN

Sitting quietly in your chosen place, bring your concentration into your breath. Don't control your breath but just pay attention as the air enters and leaves your nostrils. With each out-breath release any tension present in your physical body. Let go of all thoughts arising in your mind, visualising these as beautiful bubbles which slowly ascend into the atmosphere and then gently disperse.

When you are relaxed, visualise a shaft of clear green light coming horizontally into your body and entering your heart chakra. As the chakra becomes filled with green light it is cleansed of any emotional trauma and re-energised. When you are ready, and with the next breath, allow the green light to flow from your heart chakra into your chest cavity, bringing into a state of balance your lungs, heart and thymus gland. Emotional trauma that is not acknowledged and dealt with can have a detrimental effect upon these organs. As this colour flows into your chest, be conscious of its effect upon you. Sometimes, past traumas that you have found too painful to deal with will start to surface. If this happens, look at them and then allow them to be dissolved in the green light.

Take time to observe any effect that this colour has had before slowly opening your eyes.

When you are working with colour breathing, the effect the colour has upon you may not be felt until the exercise has been practised several times. So if, at first you feel nothing, be patient and continue to practise the given techniques.

A meditative mind is silent. It is not the silence

which thought can conceive; it is not the silence

of a still evening; it is the silence when thought – with

all its images, its words and perceptions – has entirely

ceased. This meditative mind is the religious mind – the

religion that is not touched by the church, the temples
   or by chants.

The religious mind is the explosion of love. It is

this love that knows no separation. To it, far is

near. It is not the one or the many, but rather that

state of love in which all division ceases. Like beauty,

it is not of the measure of words. From this silence

alone the meditative mind acts.

(J. Krishnamurti, *Meditations*)[1]

1   Krishnamurti, J. (1980) *Meditations*. London: Victor Gollancz Ltd.

MEDITATIONS WITH THE COLOUR GREEN

A COUNTRY WALK

Sitting in your chosen place, close your eyes and imagine that you are walking in the countryside on a warm spring afternoon. The trees that line your path are adorned with their new spring attire of pale green leaves. The grass beneath your feet is springy and soft, fresh and clean as a newly laid carpet. The grey background of the surrounding fells is patterned with a subtle green tapestry of lichens and rock plants. The only audible sound is the gentle whispering of the breeze as it meanders between the leaves of the trees and the singing of the birds as they busily collect nest-building materials. Feeling the warmth of the sun upon your body instils a feeling of peace and joy.

Following the winding path through the maze of trees, you become aware of the sound of water. At first it is barely audible, but the nearer you get to its source, the louder it becomes.

On reaching the source of the sound, you find yourself standing in front of a cascading waterfall which tumbles into a bubbling brook that rambles around large and small rocks as it makes its way to a large distant lake. Exploring the waterfall you discover a shelf of rock behind it. The shelf appears perfectly dry so you scramble up to it to investigate further. Confirming that the rock shelf is dry and quite wide, you walk along it and sit down behind the cascading water. The sound is almost deafening and it makes you realise the tremendous power that water has. The reflection from the green trees and grasses as it passes through the water bathes you in a soft, pale green light. Sitting quietly, you feel the effect that this colour has upon your heart chakra, and how it gently washes away toxins and any imbalances in your body. Your eyes become relaxed and your whole being becomes re-energised.

The feeling of aloneness created by the water and the space surrounding you allows you time for inner reflection. It is an opportunity to assess your own path in life: whether or not it is the correct path; where this path is leading; and whether or not you need to change direction. During this time of quietness, insight and inspiration may be given to you. You may find answers to questions that have been puzzling you.

When you feel ready, quietly stand and walk out from under the waterfall. Carefully descend to the path and sit down beside the brook. As you do so, become aware of your own physical body sitting in your chosen place. Before resuming your day, rest quietly for a few moments, contemplating any impressions that this visualisation has given you.

LOVING ONESELF

The heart chakra is the centre where we experience love. Love has one of the highest vibratory rates, and how we experience this depends upon how open and evolved this centre is. Love can be felt at a purely physical level, either as sexual arousal or lust, but as we evolve spiritually it is transformed into an unconditional love which encompasses all things. Before reaching this state, we have first to learn to love all aspects of ourselves. When this has been achieved, we slowly start to become the unconditional love which is able to reach out, without judgement, to all beings and conditions which we encounter.

Sitting quietly in your chosen place, relax your body and still your mind.

When you feel relaxed and at peace, withdraw into yourself. Ask yourself how much you are able to love all aspects of your being. Can you love and accept your thoughts, whether they are of a positive or negative nature? Can you love your feelings, especially when they are not very harmonious? Can you love your physical body – its shape, size and any disabilities that may be present? A lot of people have been taught that it is wrong and selfish to love themselves, but if we cannot love ourselves, can we truly love anyone else? We may be able to on an intellectual level, but this love does not come from our heart centre. Self-love involves recognising that we are constantly evolving and growing to become more powerful and loving beings and realising that the universe is literally made of love. If we will just open ourselves to receive like flowers opening to the sun, then everything is possible.

As you consider these thoughts, bring your awareness into your heart centre. Visualise this as a circular space filled with pale green light. In the centre of this space lies the bud of a pale pink rose. Pink is the colour of unconditional love. As you stand before the rose bud, it opens, and streams of pale pink light of unconditional spiritual love flow from its petals. Consciously direct this pale pink light to any part or aspect of yourself that you find difficult to love. Imagine this colour dissolving any barriers which have been erected through conditioning, and that you feel are no longer relevant for you. Fill the space left by the barriers with this pale pink light – and then send the light to anyone who you are finding difficult to love unconditionally. Ask yourself why you are unable to love this person or people unconditionally and whether this attitude is, in fact, revealing aspects of yourself that need attention.

Reflect upon these thoughts before ending this visualisation.

THE FOREST

Sitting quietly in your chosen place, slowly relax your body and quieten your mind.

Now imagine yourself walking through a forest on a hot summer's day. The forest feels cool in comparison with the surrounding fields shimmering in the heat of the mid-day sun. Looking up, observe the trees' intertwining branches creating what appears to be an arch for a living cathedral. The sun's rays filtering through the tiny gaps in the foliage create shifting patterns of light on the leaf-strewn earth. The rich greens of living foliage contrast strongly with the faded greens of decaying leaves underfoot.

Nearer the heart of the forest you find a circular pool of water that is as clear and still as crystal. Sitting down at its edge you are surrounded by the various shades of green which bring your body and mind into a state of balance and relaxation. All is still and silent. Looking into the pool you see a reflection of yourself. Look at this reflection and tell it how much you love it. Say out loud, 'I love you, I love you. I love you.'

Conscious of the heat of the day, dip your feet and legs into the pool. The coolness of the water feels wonderfully refreshing. You may even wish to venture into the pool and swim in its sparkling waters. The reflection in the water of the surrounding trees bathes you in a magical, cool green light that helps to remove any toxins present in your body and to energise and motivate you. When you feel it is time to leave the pool, sit beside it for a while, reflecting upon how you feel. Think about any insights or experiences you may have had before you open your eyes and close this meditation.

CHAPTER 6

TURQUOISE

Turquoise is a colour that is not associated with any of the major chakras. Originating in France, the word means 'Turkish stone', the gem having been discovered in the mines of Turkey. The first recorded use of turquoise as an English colour name was in 1573.

The Mayan and Inca cultures revered the turquoise stone and mined it for use in their temples and in their ceremonial dress. Turquoise is the national colour of Persia and the country is the source of some of the oldest and finest turquoise gemstones, which they call *piruesh*, meaning 'joy'. Ancient Persians believed that the turquoise could 'ward off the evil eye', giving protection to their animals as well as to themselves.

Turquoise colour is derived by mixing together blue and green, and can veer towards either depending upon the percentage of blue and green used.

Turquoise represents water. Thus the name sometimes given to the colour – aqua and aquamarine. It is a cool, calming colour which is used to boost the immune system. It can be beneficial for a person whose immune system is under par, due perhaps to a previous viral or bacterial infection. It is also valuable in calming hyperactive and over-sensitive people. Turquoise works with our intuition but it is a colour that has more to do with feeling than with rational thought. Psychologically, it invites us to become immune to stressful situations and circumstances which are depleting our energy. In the aura, turquoise is seen mainly around poets, mystics and those who are developing their intuitive powers.

BREATHING IN TURQUOISE

Sitting comfortably with a straight spine and your hands resting on your thighs, start this exercise by bringing your concentration into your breath. Breathing normally, be aware of the breath as it enters and leaves your nostrils. With each exhalation feel yourself releasing any bodily tension and allow your mind to be brought into a state of stillness.

When you are ready, with your next inhalation visualise a broad beam of turquoise light entering your body through your head and extending down into your feet. Then, with each inhalation, visualise the colour intensifying until your entire body is filled with a crystalline turquoise light. Experience the colour's cooling effect and let it remove any lingering stress or tension. Allow the colour to strengthen your immune system, making you less prone to catching any viral or bacterial infections. Still permitting this colour, with each inhalation, to enter your body, now, as you exhale, visualise the turquoise extending into your aura until you are surrounded with an orb of turquoise light.

Continue with this exercise for as long as you feel comfortable. When you are ready, and before opening your eyes, take a few moments to reflect on how this exercise has affected you. Remember that when you first start to work with these exercises you may not feel any significant changes and your mind will tend to wander on to other things. But, with regular practice, your concentration will improve and you will be able to discern the effect that each of the colours has upon you. Also, as your sensitivity to colour increases, you will intuitively know which colour you need at any given time.

MEDITATIONS WITH THE COLOUR TURQUOISE
A TURQUOISE CIRCLE

For this meditation you will need to construct a turquoise circle. It can be any size that you choose. To make the circle, take a sheet of white paper and draw a circle in its centre, using a saucer, plate or compass as your guide. Colour the circle turquoise with paint or crayons, then glue it on to a piece of stiff card and cut it out.

Placing the turquoise circle comfortably in front of you, look at the colour. Try to ascertain what feelings the colour provokes in you. Ask yourself if it is a colour that you enjoy having around or if it is a colour you are indifferent to.

Closing your eyes, imagine before them a sheet of paper, a pencil and a small pot of turquoise paint. Using your imagination, take the pencil and draw a circle on the paper. Next, pick up your paintbrush and, with the turquoise paint, colour your circle, trying to visualise the colour with your inner eye. Gaze at the circle that you have imaginatively created and allow it to expand until it enfolds you in an orb of turquoise light. Experience the colour's cooling, calming effect and, in the peace and stillness, try to listen to the voice of your intuition. Does it give answers to situations for which you are seeking a solution? Are you receiving inspiration for the next step in whatever journey you are taking?

When you are ready, increase your inhalation and exhalation before gently opening your eyes. Then put the turquoise circle in a safe place for use at another time.

THE DOLPHIN

Sitting comfortably in your chosen place, relax your body and allow all the thoughts bombarding you to float out into the atmosphere where they gently disperse.

Imagine yourself standing on a sandy beach in the Caribbean. It is a very hot, sunny day and the only shade to be found is beneath the palm trees and the numerous coloured sunshades adorning the beach. Many exotic, brightly coloured birds fly overhead, their cries mingling with the sound of the waves breaking on the sea shore.

Ready for a refreshing swim, you take yourself down to the edge of the sea. You look out over the ocean and see a vast expanse of scintillating turquoise light. The coolness of the waves as they break over your feet and legs is a welcome relief from the heat of the day.

Wading out into the water until it reaches your waist, you let yourself be lifted gently into the turquoise sea of light, enjoying its cool, relaxing freshness. Swimming in the vastness of the ocean, a great sense of timeless peace and serenity floods through you.

As you float along, buoyed up by the gentle waves, you feel something nudge your side. Turning your head, you see a large grey form swimming beneath you. As it approaches, it lifts its head from the water and you find yourself looking into the face of a dolphin. It swims around you, inviting you to play. In comparison with its size and weight, it plays very gently and makes you laugh at some of its antics. As you enjoy its presence, you become conscious that it is trying to communicate with you telepathically. It is encouraging you to hold its fin because it wants to take you down into the turquoise water to show you the beautiful world in which it lives. It tells you to have no fear of drowning because it will show you how to breathe normally under water.

Holding the dolphin's fin, you are taken down into the beauty and wonder that lies beneath the water. You pass fish of all shapes, sizes and colours, reefs of coral and rocks clothed in gently swaying sea plants. Upon reaching the ocean bed, the dolphin nudges you to stand beside it. With your hand resting on its back, you watch sea urchins and crabs scuttling across the sandy floor. All is silent as you observe the never-ending movement of the creatures that live in this watery world. You feel completely detached from your own world and immune to the pressures of people and things.

Turning and looking into the dolphin's eyes, you are able to see a reflection of yourself. You become aware of the problems and tensions that you are experiencing in everyday life, but being immune to the feelings that they evoke, you are able to see ways of resolving them. In the silence you can see your life unfolding before you: you are shown the gifts that you have been given and how these can be used to help both yourself and your companions. You see the various paths that are open to you, and which of these will bring you contentment and satisfaction.

You also realise that the radiant turquoise sea light enables you to listen to your intuition and to communicate with your higher self. That divine part of us, which knows the answers to our problems, also knows the path we should take and wants to communicate with us, if only we will listen.

Feeling a slight movement from the dolphin, you know that it is time to return to your own land-based environment. Taking hold once more of the dolphin's fin, you are gradually propelled through the water's turquoise light. As your head breaks the surface, you take a deep breath and become aware of your physical body sitting in your chosen place.

As you slowly start to increase your inhalation and exhalation, you can still see the dolphin in your mind's eye, and he assures you that whenever you wish to repeat the journey, he will be waiting – waiting to take you into the silence of the turquoise sea.

WATER

Turquoise, the colour which works on our immune system, also represents water, the element which is essential to life. Our bodies are 70 per cent water, and 70 per cent of the earth's surface is covered by water. Rivers and streams can be likened to the earth's immune system. Rain replenishes the earth with plants and crops and, by filling the rivers and streams, sustains the life of the fish and other creatures that live below its surface. It is sad to witness the destructive effect of the pollution that we have introduced into this vital element – just like the destruction and disease that drinking polluted water would inflict upon our physical body.

Sitting in your chosen place, visualise yourself in mountainous country, resting by the side of a natural lake. The stillness of the air enables the lake's surface to resemble a shiny mirror which reflects the surrounding scenery. Looking into the lake, you can see a reflection of yourself. The water's clear, quiet surface allows you to observe, in great detail, the rocks, pebbles and plants which form its foundation. You are led to consider that on a stormy day the turbulence caused by wind and rain would hide the depths of the lake from view.

Returning your concentration to your own reflection, look into your eyes. These are frequently referred to as the 'mirrors of the soul'. Can they be likened to the water in the lake? When we are in turmoil and cannot find our way out of a situation, then we are unable to see our true foundation – it is obliterated by the turbulence of our thoughts and emotions. It is only when we are happy and at peace that we are able to see clearly. Then we can look into the depth of our true being, that part of us which is eternal. This eternal part is always present but, as with the bottom of the lake, we are not always able to see it.

In a few moments of silence, try to find the depth of your true being. In order to find it, we can first calm our turbulence by breathing in the turquoise light and then, when we are ready, that eternal part of us will communicate through our intuition. As you contemplate these thoughts, visualise yourself sitting in an orb of turquoise light. Then, when you feel it is appropriate, start to increase your inhalation and exhalation before opening your eyes.

CHAPTER *7*

BLUE

Blue is at the so-called 'cold' end of the spectrum with a wavelength of 440–490 nm. The modern English word blue comes from the Middle English *bleu* or *blew*, derived from the old French word *bleu*, of Germanic origin.

Blue has an historic and symbolic association with royalty, a person of royal descent traditionally being thought to have 'blue blood'. Of Spanish origin, the saying reflected an idea that the veins of aristocrats looked bluer than those of lower ancestry.

The expression 'blue-collar workers' originates from the dark-blue clothing worn by Chinese peasants and by industrial workers in the West. This colour was worn first because the dye was easily accessible, and second because it was thought that dark blue did not show dirt as easily as did many other colours.

Although blue is a colour which suits most people and therefore is frequently worn, in this respect it does have its negative aspects. The expression 'blue gown' was the name given to ladies of easy virtue, most probably because this was the colour they were made to wear when entering a 'house of correction'. Maybe the title 'blue film' and 'blue language' stemmed from the same source.

Blue, a colour of inspiration, devotion, peace, tranquillity and harmony, helps to soothe the mind. Such attributes make it a good colour for rooms set aside for therapy, relaxation or meditation. It is a colour also credited with lowering blood pressure.

Unlike red, blue creates a feeling of space. As opposed to the constriction of red, blue opens, which makes it a good colour for asthmatics. Because it possesses the qualities of peace and tranquillity, blue is an excellent colour for those suffering from stress, tension, insomnia and high blood pressure.

On a physical level blue has few negative qualities and these are confined mainly to sadness and depression. Because of its ability to give the appearance of expansion, it can create a feeling of solitude and isolation. To counteract this tendency, orange, its complementary colour, can be used. The energy that these two colours promote is one of peaceful joy or joyful peace.

THE THROAT CHAKRA

The Sanskrit name for this chakra is *Vishuddha*, meaning 'to purify'. It is located at the neck between the two clavicle bones and is connected to our sense of hearing and to the element ether. Its dominant colour is blue. Alchemists refer to ether as the mixing bowl in which the elements of the four lower chakras are formed.

Vishuddha is pictured as a circle with 16 blue petals. Within the outer circle is a downward-pointing triangle containing a small circle. This small circle represents the full moon and its symbolic association with the chakra's attributed psychic powers. It also represents its element, ether.

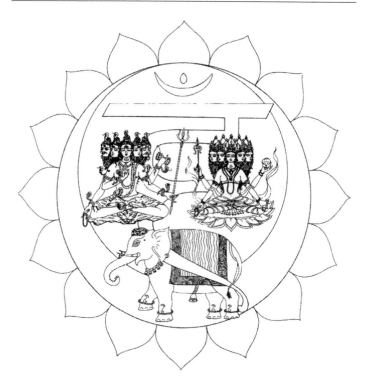

FIGURE 7.1: THE THROAT CHAKRA

Vishuddha is related to the spoken word – to sound. The sound produced at this centre is normally governed by one of the four lower chakras. If the voice is heavy and unresponsive, it comes from the earth of the base chakra; if it is soft and sexual, it comes from the sacral chakra; a warm and passionate voice belongs to the fire of the solar plexus chakra; and a gentle and sympathetic voice originates from the heart chakra.

The throat chakra forms the bridge over which we must cross to pass into the spiritual realm. It is also the bridge between the four lower elements and the principle of thought at the brow chakra.

Yogic philosophy teaches that the throat chakra is where divine nectar is tasted. This nectar is a sweet secretion produced by the lalana gland near the back of the throat. When this gland is stimulated by higher yogic practices its nectar, it is claimed, can sustain a yogi for any length of time without food or water.

On a physical level the throat chakra is associated with the nervous system, the female reproductive system, the shoulders, throat and larynx: its endocrine gland is the thyroid and parathyroids.

When this chakra has balanced energy one is well adjusted, contented and a good speaker. One may also be artistically or musically inclined. Too much energy here can lead to arrogance, self-righteousness and a dogmatic nature. A deficiency in energy can make one timid, inconsistent, unreliable and manipulative.

Some of the physical symptoms that could arise from the throat chakra are thyroid problems, weight and digestive disorders, throat problems, and pain in the neck or back of the head.

BREATHING IN BLUE

Sitting in your chosen place, gently breathe in and out for three to four minutes to a count of five, relaxing your body and quietening your mind. When you feel ready, on your next inhalation visualise a shaft of clear blue light entering the top of your head and descending into your throat chakra. As you exhale, see this colour radiating from the chakra to flood your neck before expanding out into the part of the aura surrounding it. When you feel that your throat chakra is pulsating with blue light, on your next inhalation bring the colour into your throat and, as you exhale, visualise it entering both shoulders before travelling down your arms and into your hands. Feel your shoulder muscles, your arms and hands becoming totally relaxed. If you feel tension or stress in any other part of your body, place your hands there and, still visualising this colour entering your arms and hands as you inhale, as you exhale imagine the colour leaving your hands and entering the part of the body where they have been placed. You can treat several parts of your body with blue light in this way.

When you feel ready, return to normal breathing, remaining conscious of how relaxed your body has become. This exercise can be beneficial for those working long hours at a computer, an activity which can cause a great deal of tension in the neck and shoulders.

MEDITATIONS WITH THE COLOUR BLUE

THE BLUEBELL WOOD

It is a clear, pleasantly warm day in spring and you are walking through a wood carpeted with bluebells. Finding a fallen tree trunk you sit down in order to look more closely at this splendid spectacle of colour. Observing the bluebells, you notice how gracefully and intricately they are made. Each of the tiny bells hanging from their slender green stem possesses its own individuality of colour and shape.

Closing your eyes and visualising one of these flowers, you find that its bell shape starts to expand until it completely surrounds you and you find yourself sitting inside it. The stamens provide a pillow upon which you can rest your head. Lying back you feel the petals encircling you like a soft mantle. The blue rays emanating from the petals play upon your body, releasing tension in all your muscles and organs. Your inhalation and exhalation becomes slower and gentler as your body relaxes.

In this state of relaxation you begin to contemplate the flower. The bluebell, like all other flowers, is not concerned about the future, trusting that it will be provided for. How many of us have lost this trust and, in so doing, have created for ourselves a state of tension and stress through worrying about what tomorrow will bring? Lying in the peace and tranquillity of the bluebell are you able to let go of your worries and problems, trusting that future events will take care of themselves? In doing this we learn to flow with the energies of life which will bring us to the right place at the right time, for the right purpose.

When you have thought about this and are ready to return to everyday awareness, start to increase your inhalation and exhalation, becoming aware of the bluebell shrinking back to its normal size. Become conscious of your body sitting in its chosen place then open your eyes to be ready to continue your day.

THE SKY

I have found that the most profound way of visualising blue is to contemplate the sky on a clear, sunny day.

Either visualise yourself in a sheltered and sunny place outdoors or, if possible, actually find a sheltered place outside. Lying down on the ground, look up into the vastness of the blue sky. Consider the magnitude of space and wonder whether or not it has a beginning and an ending, or whether it is infinite. How little we know about the galaxies beyond our own, and how microscopic we are in this huge cosmic field! We are like tiny droplets in a vast ocean but, as each droplet is an important part of the ocean, so we are unique and important in the great universal plan.

From looking into the sky, close your eyes and visualise the sun. Consider the important role it plays in sustaining life. Without it there would be total, lifeless darkness.

Visualise, radiating from the sun, a shaft of golden light which stretches out into the immensity of space. In your imagination, see yourself travelling along this shaft of light, out into the universe. Feel the blue light of space wrapping you in peace and protection. Listen to the sounds that each planet and star makes, and the glorious harmonies which create their symphony. Experience these sounds resonating with the sounds made by your own physical body. Each organ, muscle and bone has its own frequency; its own sound. Disharmony within the body happens when its components go out of tune – a situation which can be caused by stress, worry, diet or one's general lifestyle. Now experiment with gently humming different notes. Try to feel where these resonate within your body. See if you can find the sound that resonates with your throat chakra, the centre from which sound emanates.

Next try to visualise the vast expanse of blue sky permeating every cell of your body, releasing stress and tension and replacing these negative qualities with ones of peace and tranquillity. Immersed in that state of tranquillity, listen with your inner ear to the music of the spheres. Allow these multitudinous sounds to resonate with your physical body in order to re-tune it and restore it to harmony.

Now bring your concentration back to the colour blue, allowing it to be absorbed into your body, mind and spirit in order to create perfect peace.

When you feel ready, look for the shaft of golden light and let it carry you gently back to earth. Become aware of your physical body, feeling for any changes that may have taken place within you.

THE BRIDGE

Sitting in your chosen place, visualise yourself in the countryside on a warm spring day. Walking along a path lined with the green-leaved trees of spring, you come to a wooden bridge that crosses a peacefully flowing stream. Approaching the bridge you walk to its centre and look down into the water. Note how the water calmly flows around any obstacles that lie in its path, and listen to the restful sounds the water makes as it travels on its journey.

As you meditate upon this scene, consider your throat chakra as the bridge that takes you from a physical to a spiritual state of awareness. As we travel along life's road there are many bridges that we have to cross in order to reach the bridge at the throat centre. Take time to look at the bridges that you have crossed and what you have learnt from them. Some of these bridges may have been difficult or traumatic and some may have been easy, but reflect upon what you have learnt from each bridge that you have crossed.

Now bring your attention to your throat chakra, visualising this as the bridge that leads you to your true spiritual self. Do you feel ready to cross this bridge into a higher state of consciousness? If not, then you can stay on the bridge, wrapped in a robe of blue to give you a sense of peace and relaxation. If you choose to venture over the bridge, the only way across is through practising meditation on a regular basis. At first you may find this difficult, with your mind wandering all over the place. At this stage it is very easy to give up. But with patience and determination you will eventually glimpse the wonders that lie at the other side of the bridge and this will give you the willpower to continue – because once we glimpse something beautiful we wish to experience it more fully.

Before ending this meditation, sit quietly and assess your thoughts, ascertaining whether or not you are ready to cross the bridge of the throat chakra.

CHAPTER 8

INDIGO

The rich deep colour of indigo is obtained by combining blue and violet. This is the colour that creates space and is sometimes referred to as 'the vault of heaven on a moonless night'. In France, a moonless night was known as *l'heure bleu*, the romantic time when ladies entertained their lovers and gentlemen called on their mistresses. The colour was obtained from the indigo plant but the methods used were costly, making it almost unobtainable in the 1940s. With the introduction of synthetic dyes in the 1950s it was brought back into fashion, and became popular during the jeans revolution.

Indigo is the colour of the brow chakra, making it a good colour for fostering our intuition and for enhancing our ability to remember dreams. It helps to broaden the mind and to free it from fears and inhibitions. Because of its association with the mind, it can affect us psychically and also have a powerful effect on mental ailments. On a spiritual level, indigo represents the curtain which veils us from the light of the true spirit. When we are ready, this curtain is gently dissolved, revealing the light of the spirit and the purpose behind creation. To achieve this state, we must let go of the material world and ask to be shown how the manifest arose out of the unmanifest.

Indigo is associated with the ears and eyes, and is therefore used for some of the diseases which can affect these organs. It is also reputed to have analgesic properties, which makes it a good colour for applying to muscular aches and strains. It is also thought to be a useful colour in helping to purify the blood and the psychic currents of the aura. Being so closely related to the blue ray it can aid insomnia and help with throat-related problems.

THE BROW CHAKRA

This chakra is located between the two eyebrows at the centre of the forehead. Its Sanskrit name is *Ajna*, which is translated as 'command'. The colour radiating here is indigo. On a physical level it is affiliated to the eyes, nose, ears and brain, and the endocrine gland with which it is associated is the pituitary.

The brow chakra is depicted as two petals, symbolising our twofold nature. The challenge we are presented with here is in uniting this twofold nature to wholeness. Our twofold nature is reflected by our ego self and our spirit self; the right and left hemispheres of the brain (the intuitive and the intellectual); and our masculine and feminine energies. Yoga philosophy teaches that the base chakra contains the powerful, latent kundalini energy, referred to as the Shakti, the feminine principle. In the brow chakra resides the masculine principle, Shiva. When a person is physically, mentally, emotionally and spiritually ready, the Shakti rises through a channel in the etheric layer of the aura, known as the sashumna, which runs parallel to the physical spine, vivifying all the lower chakras on her way to the brow chakra. Here she is united with her male counterpart, Shiva, before rising into the enlightenment of the crown chakra. This symbology describes how we have to integrate both the negative and positive energies, the masculine and feminine, and the left and right hemispheres of the brain before we can complete our journey into the light of our true spiritual self.

If this chakra is out of balance, it can lead to sinus problems, catarrh, hay fever, sleeplessness, migraine, tiredness, irritability and hormonal imbalances. A hindrance to the free flow of energy to this centre is rigidity of thought, not allowing ourselves to look at other ideas and opinions and, if need be, change or modify our own.

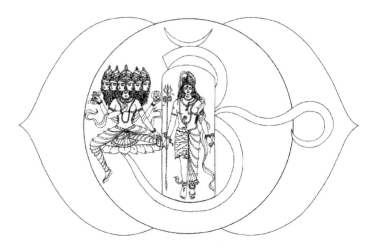

FIGURE 8.1: THE BROW CHAKRA

BREATHING IN INDIGO
ALTERNATE NOSTRIL BREATHING

Everywhere in the external world we encounter manifestations of the positive–negative principle. We find it in the composition of the atom, in the human cell, in the polarity of the earth, in the sun and moon and in the man and woman relationship. In those dimensions of existence which we gradually come to perceive through our inner vision, the same positive–negative relationship occurs. Just as we know that a certain balance must be maintained between the positive and negative in the external world, likewise a balance must be maintained in the constant interplay of positive–negative pranic current. The breathing technique that aids this is alternate nostril breathing, or *sukh purvak*, because this brings into balance the positive (the *pingala*) and negative (the *ida*) energy channels located in the etheric layer of the aura and which intertwine around the chakras, terminating at the brow chakra.

Sit either on a chair or on the floor in your chosen place. Make sure that your spine is straight and your body relaxed.

1. Place your right thumb lightly against your right nostril; your index and middle finger together on your forehead, between and just above your eyebrows, and your ring and little finger lightly against your left nostril. Extend your arm away from your body in order to allow your chest to remain open.

2. Exhale deeply through both nostrils.

3. Press the left nostril closed with the ring and little finger and inhale deeply to a count of seven through the right nostril.

4. Close the right nostril with your thumb and open the left nostril and exhale to a count of seven.

5. Repeat steps three and four for a further six times.

6. On the seventh repetition, as you inhale through your right nostril, visualise breathing in a shaft of indigo light.

7. As you exhale through your left nostril visualise this indigo light flooding your face and then extending into the aura that surrounds your head.

8. Continue working with this indigo breathing technique for as long as you feel comfortable. If at any point you feel out of breath, resume normal breathing.

ENERGISING THE FACIAL ENERGY WITH INDIGO

Sitting in your chosen place, either on the floor or on a chair, place your hands, palms down, on your thighs. Bringing your concentration to your breath, breathe normally for a few minutes in order to relax your body and mind.

When you feel ready, on your next inhalation breathe in indigo to a count of six or seven. Visualise a shaft of indigo light coming through the top of your head into your brow chakra. Exhaling to a count of six or seven, envisage this colour radiating from your brow chakra into all parts of your face and then into your aura. Continue with this technique for as long as you feel comfortable.

MEDITATIONS WITH THE COLOUR INDIGO
THE ORCHESTRA

Sitting in your chosen place, take a few moments to relax your body and quieten your mind. When you are ready, bring your awareness to your brow chakra. Visualise this chakra as a circle which then extends down into a long hall. The circular part of this hall is filled with a deep indigo light and on the floor, embossed in mosaic, is a two-petalled flower with a golden centre. Standing in the golden centre is a music conductor wearing full evening dress, with a baton in his right hand. He invites you to join him, enabling you to look down the full length of the hall. You discover that, in fact, you are looking down your physical body and your endocrine glands have become members of the orchestra.

The testes are represented by the double bass and the ovaries by the cellos. The violins and violas stand for the adrenal glands. The pancreas contains the brass section, namely the trombones, tubas, French horns and trumpets. The thymus houses the clarinets and bassoons, which are part of the woodwind section. The rest of this section, namely the flutes and oboes, depict the parathyroid and thyroid glands. Surrounding the conductor at the brow chakra are the kettledrums and cymbals and behind him, acting for the pineal gland, are the rest of the percussion section, the triangle and the tambourine.

The orchestra is ready – waiting for the conductor to give them the signal to start. He raises both his arms for quiet. Lowering his baton, he invites the orchestra to play the symphony before them. Each section renders its scripted notes which blend into an uplifting, healing, harmonious play of spectral colours.

Now the soft, pastoral section of the symphony comes into play, and with it a deep translucent indigo floods from the brow chakra to every part of this hall which represents the physical body. Great peace and stillness ensues.

Eventually the symphony ends, leaving you in a wonderful state of balance, peace and relaxation.

NIGHT

The day has passed with the last rays of the sun sinking beneath the horizon, leaving the world wrapped in the dark indigo cloak of night that is bejewelled with the glowing light from the stars. Domestic animals curl up in their baskets and kennels while farm animals bed down in their stalls or in fields beneath the night sky. The birds have returned to the trees, heads beneath their wings. The owl and other nocturnal creatures are the only souls about, hunting for food and looking for sport.

The flowers have folded their petals, encasing within them the memory of the warmth and radiance of the sun. Like the petals of the flowers, the indigo cloak of night is enfolding you within its still and tranquil energy. In this stillness, reflect upon your life, its triumphs, its mishaps, its sorrows and its joys. Take from your life's experiences its lessons and be thankful for these. Let go of all that is not relevant and therefore no longer part of you.

Reflect upon your brow chakra, from whence this colour radiates, and upon this chakra's symbolism. Take from its teaching those concepts that are right for you and leave the rest to a time when you are ready to explore further. If we plant seeds in a garden they germinate in their own time. When this time comes, we have to nurture the young seedling for it to grow into a sturdy plant. You are similar to a garden. Seeds of wisdom are planted in your fertile mind to germinate when you are ready to understand their wisdom. When this happens you have to assimilate and work with the new-found knowledge so that it may enhance your understanding of life and yourself.

Still wearing your indigo cloak of peace and protection, bring your awareness back to your physical body. Remain seated for a while, continuing to reflect upon this colour and the brow chakra's symbolism.

OUR DUALITY

The sun's rays are sinking beneath the horizon and the world is anticipating the darkness and silence of night. With the rays from the sun vanquished, the sky vibrates to the deep indigo of night, wrapping the world in a soft velvet cloak of peace and silence. Against night's indigo the stars shimmer like diamonds and the moon's halo glows with a soft orange and gold light.

Imagine that you are part of this scene and, as night gently enfolds you, all the accumulated tension, stress and strain of the past day is released. The sense of peace and feeling of relaxation allows this deep indigo to create the inner space needed for any mental or emotional pain to be dissolved.

Remember that this colour comes from your brow chakra, the centre of both physical and spiritual mind. It is the centre which is brought into play when we work with visualisation or meditation.

Concentrating on the brow chakra and its colour, try to recognise both the male and female energies within you. Are you able to accept both of these equally? Think about the intellectual and creative hemispheres of the brain. Are you integrating both of these into your life? The yin (female) and yang (male) energies are kept balanced through diet. Are you eating a well-balanced, healthy diet? It is only when we become aware of these energies that we are able to look within ourselves to discover any changes that we need to make. These changes work towards integrating our duality.

When you feel ready, bring your awareness back to everyday consciousness. Think about any changes which you need to make and then consider how these can be brought to fruition. You might find it useful to keep a personal diary of your experiences with notes on any changes that you feel you would like to make in your life. It is interesting to look back on notes you have made in order to discover if you have been able to make these changes and, if so, how they have altered your life.

CHAPTER 9

VIOLET

Violet has the shortest wavelength of all the colours and contains the highest energy. On the electromagnetic spectrum it lies next to ultraviolet, a radiation that cannot be detected by human eyes.

Violet is a mixture of red and blue but, unlike purple, with which violet is frequently confused, it has a greater proportion of blue than red. In the medieval era, manganese oxide was the pigment used to make violet stained glass. As a dye it was very expensive to produce, which meant that it could be bought only by the wealthy. This is most probably the reason why violet is associated with royalty. It is a colour also associated with luxury, very expensive jewellery often being presented in violet-lined boxes.

The earliest violet pigments used by humans, found in pre-historic cave paintings, were made from the minerals manganese and hematite. The most famous dye in the ancient world was Tyrian purple derived from a type of sea snail called the murex. During the middle ages most artists made violet by combining red taken from red ochre, cinnabar or minium, and blue taken from blue azurite or lapis-lazuli.

In nature, violet is displayed by crocuses, lavender, lilac and violets. In medieval times, violet flowers were employed medicinally, the oil extracted from them being used as a sleeping draught. Today, oil of violets is still used to flavour drinks and confectionery as well as being utilised as a perfume.

The psychological effects induced by this colour are self-respect, dignity, truth and depth of feeling. It is a colour linked with spirituality, mysticism and insight. It is also associated with modesty, hidden virtue and beauty.

Violet, comprising the vibrant energies of red and the calm, peaceful energies of blue, creates a balance between them. Because red is aligned to the masculine energy and blue to feminine energy, violet has the power to balance these two energies – energies which are found within each individual being.

The negative properties of violet are connected with introversion, decadence and suppression, and with power used for manipulation and gain.

THE CROWN CHAKRA

This chakra lies just above the crown of the head, at the end of the Sushumna nadi. It radiates the colour violet and is connected to the pineal gland. Its Sanskrit name is *Sahasrara*, which is translated as 'a thousand petalled lotus', a thousand being the number of eternity. Its petals are arranged in 20 rows and each row of 50 petals contains the 50 letters of the Sanskrit alphabet.

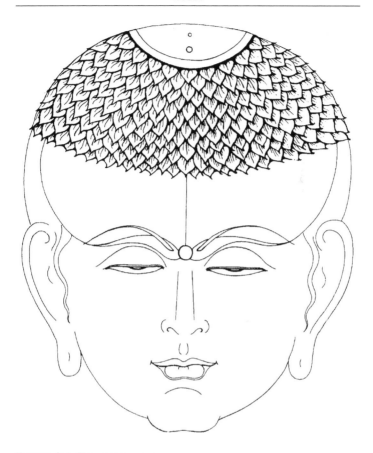

FIGURE 9.1: THE CROWN CHAKRA

This is the centre where our spiritual journey ends. Through the many challenges that life has presented and our endeavours to overcome them, we finally enter into the state of God Consciousness and become one with that ultimate reality. Our sixth sense has opened, allowing us a feeling of connectedness with both the visible and the invisible worlds. We become submerged in the vast ocean of cosmic love, peace and pure bliss. This is the state that we have worked towards through many lifetimes and the place to which all the great esoteric paths lead.

The traveller has reached the end of the journey.

In the freedom of the infinite he is free from all sorrows,

the fetters that bound him are thrown away

and the burning fever of life is no more.

In the light of his vision, he has found his freedom:

his thoughts are peace, his words are peace, his work
is peace.

(*The Dhammapada*)[1]

When the crown chakra's energy is balanced, we become
open to divine energy and have total access to the
unconscious and subconscious mind. When unbalanced,
some of the ailments that could arise are brain disease,
migraines, disorders of the endocrine system and
psychological problems.

BREATHING IN VIOLET

Sitting in your chosen place, bring your concentration
into your breath and breathe normally for five
minutes in order to relax your body and calm your
mind.

When you are ready, bring your concentration
to your crown chakra. Visualise this centre as a
lotus flower with its blossom pointing downwards.
Breathing in to a count of five to seven, visualise a
shaft of clear violet light entering the downward-
pointing lotus flower. Holding the in-breath for a
count of three, see all the lotus's petals becoming
infused with a clear violet light. Now breathe out to
a count of seven and, as you hold the out-breath for a
count of three, visualise the violet light radiating out
from the lotus into every part of your head. Continue

1   *The Dhammapada* (1972) London: Penguin Books.

this breathing sequence for five to ten minutes. Then, on the next exhalation, while holding the out-breath to a count of three, allow the violet light to radiate into the aura surrounding your head.

Continue with this exercise for as long as you feel is right for you. If at any time you become out of breath, resume normal breathing.

MEDITATIONS WITH THE COLOUR VIOLET

MEDITATION ON THE CROWN CHAKRA

Sit or lie down in your chosen place. Relax your body and quieten your mind.

In your imagination, place yourself outside the crown chakra. Slowly walk into the chakra and lie down in the centre of the violet lotus flower. You are free from all civilisation, alone and in silence.

The colour violet that radiates from this centre folds itself around you. It creates space and silent energy. It says, 'Love yourself, respect yourself, accept yourself and know that you are a microcosm of the universe.' Let go of time and space in this beautiful violet light and feel at peace with all things.

Visualise yourself as a perfect spiritual being, knowing that, if you allow yourself, you can become this being. Realise that your thoughts can influence your physical body into health or ill health, whichever you choose. Welcome the emotions and feelings that you are experiencing at this moment. Look at joy and sorrow, love and hate, comfort and pain. When you encounter negativity, change these thoughts and feelings into something that is positive. To truly love ourselves, we have to work at being positive. Initially this can prove difficult but, like all things, with practice it becomes much easier.

Be aware that your body is a temple in which is celebrated the transformation of earthly nourishment into the energies of the life-force. The spiritual energies have given unimaginable fine substances in order to allow the life-force to create seeds and plants, fruits and vegetables from which we gain this nourishment. Be thankful for this. Contemplate your diet. Are you giving your body the right nourishment for it to function at the highest possible level? Loving ourselves on all levels must encompass the way in which we think about ourselves, including the way in which we treat our physical body, the instrument in which we live.

Consider these thoughts before ending this meditation.

LOVING YOURSELF

We frequently talk about love – the love we have for a partner, husband, wife, family and friends – but how many people truly love themselves? Before starting this meditation, go and look at yourself in a mirror. Tell the reflection that you see how much you love it. You may laugh at this suggestion and feel that it is a crazy thing to do but, in spite of how you feel, try it.

Sitting in your chosen place, visualise yourself wrapped in a length of violet material. If you have a piece of material in this colour use it to wrap round yourself.

Visualising yourself clothed in violet, be aware of any feelings that this colour provokes. Ask yourself if it is a colour that you would enjoy wearing, or a colour which you dislike.

Violet is a colour which symbolises self-respect, dignity and love. What is your concept of love? Love can take many forms, be experienced on many levels, and is constantly changing until it reaches the state of ultimate love. It is at this point that a person becomes love.

Thinking about love, are you able to love yourself? Also, what is your concept of self? When this question is posed, most people identify themselves with the physical body. Perhaps this is the place where we have to start but, if we are divine beings who have no beginning and no ending and, knowing that our physical body perishes, what, then, is Divine self?

Self-love does not happen purely by luck or by the grace of God. You have to create it. So how do we begin to do this? First, pay attention to how you treat yourself compared to how you treat your friends and family. Do you beat yourself up for making a mistake or are you able to forgive yourself? Do you stay in an unhappy relationship because you are scared of being alone or can you walk away because you deserve better? Are you a door mat for others, ignoring your own needs, or do you set boundaries so that your own needs are met? Self-love will always go for the latter choices, the ones that are in your own best interest. Having said this, if you are free to act in your own self-interest you have to acknowledge everyone else's freedom to do the same thing. The difficult question is, where does self-interest end and mere selfishness begin?

Regardless of what others may think of you or say about you, every day affirm to yourself 'I love and accept myself as I am.' When you are praised, accept the praise and say thank you.

Keeping your eyes closed, bring your awareness back to your violet cloaked physical body. Endeavour to visualise the colour. Imagine violet interacting with your physical body, saturating every molecule and atom and suffusing you with respect and dignity. Allow this colour to extend into your emotions and intellect, thereby teaching you to respect your feelings and thoughts.

Before ending this meditation, sit for a while in silence, considering what you have experienced with this colour and what this meditation has taught you.

THE CRYSTAL ROOM

A crystal that reflects the colour violet is the amethyst. Its name comes from the Greek word *amethustos*, meaning 'without drunkenness'.

Amethyst is a powerful healing stone and is found in light and dark violet shades. The lighter shades can be used for mysticism and spiritual inspiration, whereas the darker ones act as powerful transformers of energy. The amethyst is a stone of inspiration and humility, reflecting the love of God. It is a wonderful stone to use in healing, especially in conjunction with colour healing. It helps both emotional and physical pain.

Sitting in your chosen place, gradually start to relax your body and quieten your mind. Visualise the thoughts entering your mind as beautiful bubbles which lightly float into the atmosphere and disperse.

Visualise yourself standing beside a giant amethyst crystal. Walking around the crystal you discover a door in one of its facets. This door has a round crystal handle on its left side. Take hold of the handle and turn it; push the door open and walk through into a crystal room. The floor of this room is covered with a deep violet carpet.

After closing the door, walk to the centre of the room. Sitting or lying down on the carpet, you discover that the room is bathed in a soft violet light which restfully gathers around you. You start to feel the life-force that permeates the crystal and the quiet, almost inaudible sound to which it vibrates. As these sensations start to interact with your physical body you find yourself encapsulated in an orb of love and light. All the emotional pains and traumas that have been part of your life melt peacefully away and are replaced with the vibrational force of spiritual love. This enables you to look with love at all aspects of yourself, and creates the necessary space for you to be able to break, and let go of, all the emotional ties which you feel are no longer beneficial to you. With love, submit these ties to the soft violet light of the amethyst. Watch them being gently dissolved in order that they can be re-formed to a higher level of understanding. This action perfects within you a feeling of lightness, joy and well-being.

With these new-found feelings integrating into your everyday life, it is time to leave your crystal room and return to your daily tasks. Rising from the floor or chair, walk back to the crystal door. Turn the handle and pull open the door. Walk through, closing the door behind you, back to the place where you chose to practise this meditation. Before opening your eyes, take time to consider what this meditation may have helped you to realise about yourself.

CHAPTER 10

MAGENTA

The colour magenta is a combination of red and violet. If we view a rainbow in its three-dimensional form, where the red and the violet meet, magenta is created.

The magenta dye was first produced by the French, who called it *fuchsine* after the fuchsia plant. It was renamed magenta by the Italians after one of their villages, near which an especially bloody Franco-Prussian battle was fought.

In fashion, this colour overtook violet in popularity during the latter half of the nineteenth century. In the 1960s magenta was used in conjunction with orange to make what was referred to as a 'psychedelic' vibration. This symbolised ringing the changes and defying existing rules and regulations. In the 1930s, a bright, intense magenta was called 'shocking pink', in the 1950s it was 'hot pink' and in the 1960s 'kinky pink'.

On a physical, emotional and mental level, magenta is the colour of 'letting go', in order that change may take place. It assists us in letting go of old thought patterns born from conditioning, releasing old emotions which live in the past, and giving up physical pursuits which we have outgrown. When we are able to do this, we free ourselves to flow with the tide of life. Only then can change necessary for our spiritual growth take place.

Magenta represents universal love at its highest level. It promotes cooperation, kindness, compassion and encourages a sense of self-respect in those who use it. It is a cheerful and happy colour and helps us to appreciate all that we have achieved in life.

Its negative aspects are its ability to promote depression and despair in some people and, in others, to prevent them from meeting any challenges with which they are faced. Too much magenta can generate arrogance and make us intolerant of others.

BREATHING IN MAGENTA

Sitting comfortably in your chosen place, make sure that your spine is straight and your body relaxed. Start this exercise by taking a few deep breaths through your nose to quieten your mind and to totally relax your body.

When you feel ready, bring your awareness to your physical body, visualising this as an empty vessel – but be conscious of one of the body's largest organs, your skin.

Next, breathing in to a count of eight, visualise a shaft of white light entering through the top of your head and filling your inner space. As you breathe out visualise, as a grey mist, any negativity, any past traumas, and any discomfort that your body may be holding being released through your nose and through all the pores in your skin. Continue to do this until you feel that all negativity has been released.

On your next in-breath, visualise a shaft of magenta light entering through the top of your head and filling the whole of your being. Allow this light to make any changes that are physically, emotionally and mentally necessary to bring you into optimum health. As you exhale, watch this magenta light flow out of your body through the pores in your skin and into your aura to strengthen and vivify it. Continue to inhale and exhale this magenta light for five to ten minutes, becoming conscious that with each breath energy is building up within you. Then, when you are ready to finish this breathing exercise, take a few moments to ascertain how you are feeling. With practice, you can increase the length of time taken for any of the breathing exercises given.

MEDITATIONS WITH THE COLOUR MAGENTA

SUNSET

Going to your chosen place, relax your body and quieten your mind.

Visualise yourself sitting on a hilltop at sunset. The last rays of the sun create a spread of magenta across the sky. Looking at this wonderful spectacle of colour enables you to let go and just 'be'. Time and space dissolve, creating within you a void which enables you to look more clearly at yourself. Watching the colour pageant which is unfolding around you, you enter into a state of silence and peace. As you gaze at the magenta that now dominates the sky, this colour comes and enfolds you, enabling you to see yourself as you are in this moment of time. It also allows you to see yourself in a perfected state. You ask: 'How do I obtain this state of perfection?' The answer you intuitively receive is: 'Let go; let go of all things that are no longer right for you and which prevent you from attaining this state that you desire; let go, in order that you may flow with the energies of life.' Inwardly you know that the answer given is correct, but initially it creates in you fear and insecurity. Perhaps the first stage in this process is, at the end of each day, to review the day in order to discover anything that you need to change or work with – but also to praise yourself for all that you have achieved. The next stage is to begin to let go of your fear and insecurity, knowing that all change can be uncomfortable but, once achieved, can be very rewarding. Try to look upon your fears and insecurities as stepping stones towards the image of your perfected self.

Meditating upon these thoughts, watch as the sun sinks beneath the horizon and the magenta sky turns into the deep indigo of night, cloaking you in a robe of peace and security. Then, when you are ready, increase your inhalation and exhalation before slowly opening your eyes.

GRATITUDE

For this meditation you will need a magenta-coloured rose. If you are unable to obtain one, then recall from your memory an image of this magenta flower.

For many people the rose conjures up a picture of a country cottage garden. Roses are given for birthdays, anniversaries and to say thank you. Red roses are associated with love and affection, while the magenta rose is identified with spiritual love.

Sitting in your chosen place, if you have managed to obtain a magenta rose hold it in your hands and meditate upon it. If you have been unable to find one, then close your eyes and imagine this magenta flower before your closed eyes.

Marvel at the way in which the tight bud has unfolded into what appears to be a spiral of petals. Notice how the sepals, which covered and protected the bud, have fallen away and lie drooping against the stem. Discover how each petal is formed and its overall varying magenta shades. Observe how, when light falls upon the rose, it creates areas of darkness and light. Look at the centre of the flower in order to discover what lies there.

From the blossom, look at or visualise the stem and leaves of the rose. Note the thorns that grow on its stem, forming a layer of protection. If you are working with a live rose, you will find that its leaves are also prickly to the touch. In contemplating the leaves, do you find that they in any way resemble the petals?

If you are not already working with closed eyes, close them and try to visualise the rose. Does this flower remind you of all the glorious warm days and balmy nights of summer? Does it recall any happy events of summers past? In order to work with eradicating from your life those things to which you no longer resonate, so that you can evolve as a spiritual being, first look with gratitude at all the blessings that you have received; at the gifts that you have been given and the love of your friends and family. Recall all the positive things that have happened to you and be truly grateful for these. Then look at things that you feel you need to change. Perhaps you are being unkind to yourself in letting people use you for their own gain. If this is true, ask yourself why you are allowing this to happen. Is it because you want to be loved and needed by others? If so, first start by loving yourself. You also need to learn how to say one very simple, small word – and that word is NO. Sometimes, allowing others to use us stems from childhood conditioning when we were taught that it is selfish to think of ourselves first. Remember, if we are unable to care for ourselves, eventually we will not be able to care for anyone else because our strength and life-force will have been drained from us.

After meditating upon these thoughts, visualise this magenta rose at the centre of your heart chakra. Envisage shafts of pale magenta light flowing from the tips of its petals into your body and then extending beyond your body into your aura and then into the room where you are sitting. Visualise this room becoming filled with a pale magenta light which changes the room's vibration into one of pure love. Visualise anyone who enters this room being touched by, and experiencing, the wonderful atmosphere that has been created by this colour.

When you feel ready, gradually increase your inhalation and exhalation before opening your eyes.

Having offered meditations on the eight colours of the spectrum, this book ends with a meditation encompassing the complete spectrum and allows you, the reader, to choose, experience and work with the colour you feel most attracted towards.

THE NIGHT SKY

Sitting in your chosen place, relax and gently close your eyes.

Imagine that you are lying in the middle of a field on a warm summer's night. Looking into the night sky, you perceive it as a large, orbicular bowl of deep indigo light studded with clusters of lustrous, sparkling stars. As you meditate upon this scene, time and space stand still, allowing you to travel into and become part of the picture. The deep colour of indigo protects you and enfolds you in a feeling of peace and contentment as your journey takes you to the edge of what appears to be the brightest star. The brilliant white light radiating from this star forms a tunnel for you to stroll down. Walking to the end of the tunnel, you encounter a wonderful sight. The white light from the star has fragmented into the eight colours of the spectrum. Nearest to you, on your right-hand side, is red, the colour of energy, warmth and vibrancy, a colour that helps to keep you grounded. By its side is orange, which lifts your spirits and helps you to enjoy all the good things that life has to offer, making you want to laugh and dance along your chosen path. Next comes yellow, a colour which helps you to work with your intellect and aids you in stepping back from stressful situations, thus making it easier to find the right solution. From yellow we come to the soothing colour of green, a colour that brings harmony and balance to your bodily systems and to your thoughts and emotions. Moving away from green we reach blue, the colour of peace and relaxation, one which can slow down our metabolism and lower blood pressure. Adjacent to blue is indigo, a colour which creates space for those things which we wish to pursue and helps to ease our physical, emotional or mental pain. Indigo is followed by violet, a colour connected with divinity and royalty but which also helps us to respect and appreciate ourselves. Finally we arrive at magenta, the colour that helps us to make the changes necessary for our evolution as spiritual beings.

After observing and digesting this panoply of colour, choose and walk into the colour that you feel attracted towards. Ask yourself why you have chosen this colour then allow it to surround and interpenetrate your physical body. When you feel ready, walk out of your chosen colour, back through the tunnel of light, until you reach the place where you started this meditation. Take a few moments to contemplate the meditation's effect upon you before opening your eyes.

EPILOGUE

Now that you have looked through this book, you will have seen that there are several ways of discovering the colour that will be most beneficial for you. You may intuitively know the colour. If not, then you can either make yourself a colour wheel containing the colours discussed in the book and then use the wheel to dowse for your colour (see page 28), or you can obtain a set of coloured materials, place these either on a table or on the floor, and then choose the colour that you feel drawn towards. When working in this way, you may find that the same colour comes up for you on several consecutive days. If this happens, choose to work with a different meditation for that colour on each consecutive day.

I would recommend that you keep a diary of your work with colour and meditation. A record of what you have discovered about yourself can be very useful. You might also find it helpful to mention how each colour has affected you at different times. If you feel that certain colours are detrimental to you, don't stop working with them: it may well be that their effect on you was needed to bring your being back into a state of wholeness. Remember that if we are unwell we are off colour, and introducing the correct colour or colours back into the body can sometimes be uncomfortable not just physically but, at times, emotionally and mentally.

When working with meditation, you may find that you start to remember your dreams more clearly. If possible, have a note book and pen by your bed to write down your dream immediately upon waking: dreams can tell us a great deal about ourselves, but they have a habit of fading from memory very rapidly!

If you are a very sensitive person, it is advisable to close down your chakras after each meditation. The easiest way of doing this is to visualise them as beautiful lotus flowers: then, starting with the crown chakra and working down to the base chakra, visualise each lotus flower closing back to a bud.

We began our rainbow journey by considering the importance of light – light which encompasses all the colours of the spectrum, beginning with red and finishing with magenta – the colour which brings us full circle and takes us into another space and another kind of light.

If we view the rainbow in its three-dimensional form, it creates a circle where the red and violet join to create magenta. Magenta is the colour of change, change which can lift us into a higher dimension or allow us to step up onto the next rung of the ladder, allowing us to see the life-path which we have chosen to follow from a different perspective. From this point we are able to see the rainbow's more ethereal colours, colours which appear in more subtle shades and vibrate to a higher frequency. Having reached this stage in our journey prepares us to meditate with each of these subtle shades until we again reach the translucent colour of magenta which contains within it the pale pink of unconditional love. Here again we can make a quantum shift to our next level of awareness. This progression into ever higher states of consciousness continues until we reach that state of God consciousness where we are able to answer the much asked question 'Who am I?', and find ourselves enfolded in the inexpressible light of eternity.

Thank you for accompanying me on this rainbow journey, and I hope that you will enjoy working with this book as much as I have enjoyed writing it.

INDEX

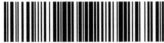

Made in the USA
Middletown, DE
13 January 2019